KIDS &
DRUGS

KIDS &
DRUGS
A PARENT'S HANDBOOK OF DRUG ABUSE PREVENTION & TREATMENT

Jason D. Baron, M.D.
Founder, Drug Abuse Programs of America

A GD/PERIGEE BOOK

For Sallye, Adam, Andy, and Beau
Love is always close to me

Perigee Books
are published by
The Putnam Publishing Group
200 Madison Avenue
New York, New York 10016

Library of Congress Cataloging in Publication Data

Baron, Jason D.
  Kids and drugs.

  Bibliography: p.
  Includes index.
  1. Drug abuse.   2. Children—Drug use.   3. Parent and
child.   I. Title.   [DNLM: 1. Substance abuse—In adolescence—Handbooks.   2. Substance abuse—Therapy—Handbooks.   WM 270 B265k]
RC564.B36   1983   362.2'9386   83-11390
ISBN 0-399-50847-3

First Perigee Printing, 1984

Printed in the United States of America

1 2 3 4 5 6 7 8 9

Acknowledgments

I wish to express my gratitude and appreciation to the
many people who have encouraged and aided me in the
completion of this book.

The enthusiasm and optimism of parent groups around
the country, and in particular that of Peggy Mann, was of
great support. The staff of DAPA was a source of
inestimable value. Advice and comments from therapists,
counselors, nurses, and ancillary departments showed a
cohesiveness of thought and practice that I hope is
evident in the chapter on treatment.

I wish to also thank my staff—Donna Morris, Sandy
Lackey, Pattie Wolfe, and Russell Morris—for their
untiring efforts to gather material, offer suggestions,
complete the manuscript, and work beyond what was
expected to complete this project.

Mostly I would like to thank my wife, Sallye, for her
constant support, reassurance, and love during the
preparation of this handbook. She freely gave up many
nights and weekends to be there when I needed her.

—JASON D. BARON, M.D.

Contents

Preface

I first became aware of the enormous drug epidemic when I joined the National Institute of Mental Health in 1968. During my two years at the Clinical Research Center for Drug Addiction, which is part of NIMH, I saw hundreds of heroin addicts hospitalized for severe drug addiction. Hardly any of them had begun their drug abuse with heroin—they progressed to it from "soft drugs."

Since the opening of my hospital drug-abuse program in 1975, some nine thousand patients have been treated by our staff. As the age of our younger patients steadily decreased, I became more concerned about the spread of drugs throughout America. As a psychiatrist specializing in child and adolescent behavior and drug and alcohol abuse, I was able to see firsthand the horrible stresses that a family endures when their youngsters begin to use drugs.

In the most recent years of my practice, I have become increasingly aware of a vast vacuum of literature for parents concerned about preventing drug abuse in their children. In addition, little material is available for parents who want to know about the treatment of the drug-using adolescent and adult.

It is my hope that this book will stimulate parents to become actively involved in drug-abuse prevention early in the lives of their children. Much of the information in Chapter 2, Prevention, is currently being used by a number of parent peer groups across the country. I have attempted to incorporate their experiences, advice, and efforts into a step-by-step guide for the organization of parent peer groups.

Chapter 3, Treatment, is intended to present a hospital in-patient program in some detail. I hope to enlighten parents about the specific types of treatment that are available, explain the direct effects of these therapies, and provide a checklist for evaluating a hospitalization program. The discussion of community drug-abuse programs is also of importance because much of the success of a hospital program is dependent on continued treatment in an effective after-care program.

Any suggestions, advice, or comments from the readers of this book would be greatly appreciated. I believe that we can reverse the escalating spread of drug abuse in America by sharing ideas, examining new techniques, and using our creative potential to the fullest.

This book includes material about a number of commonly abused drugs. Although many parents are most interested in marijuana, I know from my experience that most teenagers begin their experimentation with either marijuana or alcohol and move on to other drugs. Relatively few of these teenagers do not experiment with other drugs. In some cases this may take years to occur; in others it happens within a few weeks to months. The drugs teens try most frequently or use regularly include alcohol, stimulants (amphetamines and cocaine), depressants (barbiturates, Quaaludes, Mandrax, Valium, and Librium), hallucinogens (LSD, PCP, peyote, etc.), inhalants, and opium and its derivatives. In a recent survey of 2000 charts of teenagers between the ages of twelve and nineteen, I found only 94 who had used *only* marijuana. This means that over 95 percent of the patients I have treated had a history of "poly-drug" use. This figure is probably not true for the general population, but it is significant enough to warrant parent education about the other commonly abused drugs besides marijuana.

1

The Drugs

Ricky J. missed his first appointment with me. His parents came instead, furious about their sixteen-year-old's behavior and feeling hopeless. They had told Ricky the night before that they had arranged an interview with a psychiatrist, and he had become angry, verbally abusive, and finally walked out of the house. They had not heard from him since 7 P.M. the previous evening and had been up most of the night worrying about him.

Ricky's parents related a story that I have heard literally thousands of times. Their son had a normal childhood, had many friends, was lovable, intelligent, and considerate until about age thirteen. At that point he began to replace his old friends with new ones, showed increasing signs of irritability, anger, disregard for feelings of family members, apathy, and loss of interest.

The situation had been steadily worsening. Ricky was viewed by other parents as being a bad influence for their children, and they refused to allow him to visit. Frequent discipline and truancy problems emerged. His grades fell precipitously at age fourteen, and he no longer showed any interest in schoolwork. He began to withdraw from the whole family and to "explode" verbally when any limits or rules were enforced. He locked his room whenever he was at home and refused to let his parents in.

Eventually his parents discovered his use of marijuana. They found rolling papers and marijuana pipes hidden in his room and in the garage. When they confronted him, he told them that "all the kids do it." He felt it caused no change in his life and was determined to continue using it whenever he felt like it. He denied using any other drugs, including alcohol.

Ricky did return home. He was in his room when his parents returned from their appointment with me. At this point his father blew up at him. His own nerves and those of his wife were strained. After pleading with Ricky to go with them for an evaluation, and being refused, Mr. J. told Ricky to pack some clothes and leave home. Basically Ricky knew he could not cope with street life, so he reluctantly agreed to see me.

At this session Ricky had a know-it-all, rebellious attitude toward me, the drug-abuse program, and his parents. After talking privately with me and realizing that his parents would not allow him to return home without treatment, he agreed to enter a hospital treatment program. On entering the hospital, his urine and blood drug screens showed only marijuana. He was smoking two to three joints per day, rarely more.

The type of treatment Ricky received is detailed in Chapter 3. The treatment was successful. Ricky and his parents are now active in a community drug-abuse program, and the family no longer fits the description of a family in crisis.

Because marijuana is used by so many millions of adolescents and young adults, the first chapter of this handbook will review some of the findings presented by marijuana researchers. Many of us in the drug-abuse prevention and treatment fields feel that marijuana is a "gateway" drug—a drug that opens the door to further experimentation with more drugs. A description of other drugs teenagers commonly use follows.

CANNABIS SATIVA
marijuana, hashish, hash oil, THC

MARIJUANA

Parent groups are attempting to educate the public about marijuana, as it is the drug most frequently tried by preteens and teenagers. The parents feel that if marijuana use can be prevented, then a teenager is less likely to use the other drugs that are available in our neighborhoods and cities.

Most parent groups interested in drug-abuse prevention are familiar with the large amount of literature about marijuana that has resulted from various research programs. Four of the more outstanding scientists in the field are Dr. Carlton Turner (director of the National Institute on Drug Abuse Research Project on Marijuana), Dr. Gabriel Nahas (Columbia University), Dr. Robert Heath (Tulane Department of Psychiatry), and Dr. Ethel Sassenrath (U.C.–Davis Primate Research Center). These experts and a vast number of others have published over 7500 studies on the medical and psychological effects of marijuana that counter the widespread myth that marijuana is a harmless drug. This inaccurate information originated in the 1960s. At that time only a very weak grade of marijuana with a THC content of only about 0.5 percent was available. THC (delta-9-tetrahydrocannabinol) is the psychoactive ingredient in marijuana. THC is only one of the 420-odd chemicals that have been isolated from marijuana.

During the 1970s and 1980s marijuana has become a very different drug from what it was in the 1960s. In addition to its vast availability, the THC content is much, much higher. Marijuana strains have been refined, and strengthened in the process, to produce a drug that has a more powerful effect on the user. Many strains are available with a THC content of over 5 percent, thus making marijuana at least ten times as powerful as it was during the 1960s. Some of the common stronger strains are known as Sinsemilla, Colombian, and Acapulco Gold. Other common names for marijuana are: dope, ganja, hemp, joint, maryjane, pot, reefer, roach, and weed. Many locales have their own idiomatic slang for marijuana.

Marijuana comes from the hemp plant *Cannabis sativa,* a hardy weed that can grow in most climates. It is difficult to eradicate and is grown in many states, especially California and Hawaii. It can be grown in large gardens or mixed in with other plants to avoid detection. Mexico, Colombia, and other Latin American countries grow an enormous crop yearly.

During recent years marijuana growing has become big business in the United States. Crops in California have become the leading agricultural product in many counties, bringing in millions of dollars annually to unscrupulous farmers. The same is true in Hawaii. The government's latest projection of estimated sales in the United States was, conservatively, $48 billion, making marijuana production the third largest industry in America.

The user of marijuana buys "grass" in small plastic bags usually containing one ounce, or a "lid." The price of a lid varies from $40 to even $200 according to locale, grade of marijuana, and the supply available. A middleman buys large quantities from the grower, divides it into smaller parcels, and may sell directly to the user or to another middleman, who in turn sells to the small purchaser.

The buyer on the street usually receives it as a mixture of chopped leaves, stems, twigs, seeds, and flowers. The seeds can be replanted in yards or grown as indoor plants.

Most lids are "cleaned" after purchase, the seeds taken out for planting and the stems and twigs brewed into a tea. The flowers contain the greatest amount of THC.

Commercial cleaners are sold via mail order from pro-drug magazines or can be purchased in "head shops" (drug paraphernalia stores). The cleaned marijuana is usually rolled into a "joint" by using cigarette rolling papers purchased from convenience, drug, and grocery stores. The final product is a joint that resembles a thin cigarette.

Marijuana smoke is abrasive, and many people use a water pipe to inhale it. The smoke passes through water in the pipe and is rendered less harsh and irritating in this manner. Another favorite is a "carburetor" or a "bong," which allows a large amount of marijuana smoke to be collected in this glass container, then forcefully inhaled deep into the lungs to maximize the amount inhaled.

As a joint is smoked it becomes too small to hold. At this point it is termed a "roach," and "roach clips" are sold in a variety of sizes and shapes. Most are basically alligator clips attached to holders. With this device a user can smoke all of a joint without burning his fingers.

Another method of ingestion is eating marijuana. Usually it is strained to a fine powder and sprinkled on salads or cooked in brownies. It has an unappetizing taste if eaten raw and can cause nausea.

If parents find any of this paraphernalia among their child's belongings, there is an excellent chance that marijuana is being used, probably frequently. Parents should never hesitate to examine their children's rooms if drug use is suspected—it is possible to stop abuse at an early stage if it is discovered.

Another thing to be aware of about marijuana and its controversial harmful side effects is the "Jamaican Study." This study, which is quoted by many prodrug groups as proof that marijuana is a "safe" drug, has been consistently disputed by the scientific community, and although many prodrug groups present it as fact, is quite obviously a poorly designed study that is being used politically in an attempt to legalize a harmful drug. The study was done in 1972, and, as in the 1960s, the grade of marijuana used was weak. The results were inconclusive. To date, thousands of scientific publications point to a multitude of dangerous effects of marijuana, and *no* scientific journal to my knowledge has agreed to publish the Jamaican Study as a valid scientific article.

In summarizing some of the effects that have been found by scientific research over the last few years, I will mention some highlights, but I refer you to *Marijuana: An Annotated Bibliography,* Volume 1, by Dr. Carlton Turner and his associates (Macmillan Information, 200-D Brown St., Riverside N.J., $14.95) for a detailed listing of literature.

Evidence shows that marijuana is a fat-soluble chemical. This means that once marijuana is present in the body, it becomes stored in the fat cells and is not excreted rapidly by urine and sweat, as is alcohol. The half-life (time for one-half of the material to be excreted) is seventy-two hours. All of it is not excreted for approximately twenty-one days. Therefore, if one smokes marijuana more frequently than once every three weeks, it is being accumulated and stored in the fat cells. This is not to say that one has the "euphoric" high for this period, but rather that the marijuana chemicals (some 420 extraneous chemicals) are present in the body.

The scientific evidence shows that these chemicals affect every organ system in the body. Dr. Robert Heath of Tulane Medical School has proved the existence of cholesterol deposits in the brains of rhesus monkeys following ingestion of THC alone. This impairs the electrical circuits of the brain. In other words, the brain cells cannot communicate with the other brain cells. This may be the reason why the person high on pot often forgets what he is saying in mid-sentence.

Many researchers feel that if marijuana is used over a period of time, the brain-cell alterations may be irreversible. This is because the brain consists largely of fat, and marijuana has a propensity to store itself in fat cells.

Dr. Heath demonstrated clearly that active marijuana smoking in rats led to irreversible alterations in brain functions after just three months. Many psychiatrists have noted a definite personality change in marijuana users, who often show apathy, lack of motivation, hostility, anger, and resentment.

There is much agreement that heavy marijuana use can result in brain atrophy, especially in the cerebrum, the "thinking" part of the brain. The results of a study conducted by Dr. I. R. Rosengard, involving 37,000 subjects, suggested that regular use of marijuana produced cerebral atrophy (shrinking of the cerebrum) in young adults.

Documented research conducted throughout the country suggests chemical changes (deficiencies in brain protein and RNA), acute brain syndromes (clouding of mental thinking, disorientation, memory impairment, confusion), retardation of normal development, and production of abnormal thinking patterns (misperceptions, illusions, delusions, irritabilities, anxieties, aggressiveness, and distortion in perception of time, space, and sound).

Marijuana does not affect only the brain. Other systems that are involved include the respiratory, reproductive, sensory, hepatic (liver), cardiac (heart), and lymphatic (glands); and marijuana is known to produce a host of psychological and emotional changes.

One of the most significantly affected systems is the reproductive system—a system that is high in fat content. Tests conducted by my staff as well as other researchers show that daily marijuana smoking causes a lowering of testosterone, the male sex hormone. Testosterone levels need to be of normal values in young males so that the body can mature in the areas of muscle growth, hair distribution, genital size, bone size and strength, and sperm production.

Without these normal levels, sperm count and sperm motility can be reduced, and sexual dysfunction and impotence may result.

Marijuana's effects on the young female are also startling. Researchers have found serious abnormalities in the rhesus monkey, an animal with a menstrual cycle similar to that of the human female (Dr. Ethel Sassenrath, U.C.–Davis Primate Center). Ovulation and lactation are interfered with, and the number of stillborns is increased fourfold. The genetic effects on babies is unknown, but many scientists feel that subtle congenital abnormalities may exist. The testosterone level in females is increased, as opposed to the decrease in males. In general, *any* drug that interferes with these normal hormonal changes in an adolescent girl may interfere with her ability to have a normal reproductive development.

There are studies that show that marijuana alters vision, causes reddening of the eyes by action on the blood vessels in the conjunctiva, affects sight and hearing, and produces severe irritation of the throat.

There is also a definite link with cancer. Precancerous cells have been shown to result from marijuana smoking, and many researchers feel it is definitely cancer causing. Respiratory impairments include marked bronchitis, emphysema, pharyngitis, asthma, nasal inflammation, reduction in pulmonary function tests, laryngitis, and hoarseness. Furthermore, smoking marijuana also weakens the body's natural resistance to infectious diseases by paralyzing the alveolar macrophages (one of the body's first lines of defense).

There is evidence of microsomal changes in the liver, reducing the body's ability to decompose toxic material, and signs of liver degeneration. Other medical findings—actually thousands of reports—verify the physical effects that marijuana has on the body.

Even more clear are the psychological effects. Parents of

teenagers already using pot will be familiar with most if not all of the following signs and symptoms. Most of these symptoms apply to all the drugs in this chapter.

PHYSICAL SYMPTOMS

1. Change in activity level—periods of lethargy or fatigue (common with marijuana, alcohol, sedatives, cocaine, heroin, and PCP) and periods of hyperactivity (common with marijuana, amphetamines and other stimulants, and alcohol).
2. Change in appetite varying from increase to decrease and cravings of certain foods (sweets are common with marijuana). Increase or decrease in weight.
3. Lack of coordination—staggering gait, slow movements, dropping objects, clumsiness, falling.
4. Altered speech patterns—slurred or garbled speech, flat or expressionless speech, pressured speech (fast talking), forgetting thoughts and ideas, incomplete sentences.
5. Shortness of breath, hacking cough, peculiar odor to breath and clothes (often with marijuana).
6. Red eyes, watery eyes, droop to eyelids.
7. Runny nose, increased susceptibility to infections and colds.
8. Change in sleeping habits—staying up all night, sleeping all day, insomnia, excess sleeping, refusal to wake up.
9. Change in appearance—change in style of clothes, less concern about appearance, which may become sloppy and unkempt.
10. Severe agitation, lack of concentration, shaking, tremors of extremities, nausea, vomiting, sweats, chills (may be an early withdrawal syndrome from drugs).
11. Distortion of perception of time—short times may feel much longer; reaction time becomes sluggish.
12. "Needle tracks"—which may occasion wearing long-sleeve shirts in all weather to hide needle marks from intravenous injection of drugs. Tracks may be in hidden areas, such as the back of legs. Absence of tracks does not preclude drug abuse or addiction.

SOCIAL AND EMOTIONAL CHANGES

1. Mood alteration—changes and "swings" in mood—from euphoria and gregariousness to irritability, anxiety, violence, bizarreness, depressed mood, outbursts of anger.
2. Thought-pattern alterations—lack of thoughts, strange and bizarre thinking, hallucinations, paranoid delusions, suspiciousness, depressed thoughts, suicidal thoughts.
3. Withdrawal, secretiveness, deviousness, vagueness, hypersensitivity, placing the room off-limits to family.
4. Sudden changes in friends, disdain for old friends, new people calling, frequenting new hangouts, people stopping by for very short periods.
5. Drop in school performance, truancy, resentment toward teachers, avoiding schoolwork (or not bringing books home), lack of interest and concentration span in school and generally ("amotivational syndrome").
6. New idols, especially drug-using rock stars, songs with drug lyrics, older kids.
7. Legal problems—late hours, traffic violations, assaultiveness, disrespect for police, eventually possession of paraphernalia and drugs.
8. Resentment toward all authority.
9. Presence of paraphernalia, incense, room deodorizer, eyedrop bottles, seeds, and drugs.
10. Flagrant disregard for all rules—school, home, legal.

With marijuana use, there is an enormous change in the user's memory, both long- and short-term. Most parents note this, and the research confirms it. Not only do drugs affect short-term, long-term, and immediate memory function, they also interfere in the process of transfer between the memory functions.

Sense of time is another function that is altered, causing problems with normal reflexes. If a person is high and asked to raise his hand when one minute has elapsed, he usually does so in ten to fifteen seconds. There is no doubt that being high on marijuana or other drugs is the cause for a very large proportion of accidents and fatal car wrecks.

Additionally, learning impairment is almost always present with frequent usage. I can usually tell when marijuana smoking has become a daily pattern by reviewing a student's transcript. Grades begin to fall precipitously in almost all cases. Thinking is not clear, and the selection of extraneous material to be incorporated into one's internal thought process is faulty. The speed of performing tasks is altered, even such simple thinking as arithmetic or copying figures. Larger, frequent doses begin to affect logical thinking.

Thought processes are gradually changed from continued usage. Just some of the alterations include a blurring of past and present experiences; a sense of timelessness; periods of well-being vacillating with periods of moodiness, anxiety, panic, fear, depersonalization, and depression. Psychotic thinking is easily precipitated in emotionally unstable users or in those under great stress. More and more recent studies indicate increasing numbers of users who develop illusions, paranoid delusions, and hallucinations. Some people report a loss of the sense of reality.

Many of these severe reactions have occurred because people are using a kind of marijuana that is really a different drug from the marijuana of the 1960s. As its potency increased, so did its side effects. It is impossible for the average person to know the grade or potency of the drug he or she is buying; only smoking it will reveal how strong it is.

To further complicate the situation, weaker marijuana is often adulterated with chemicals to give it more "kick." A frequently used addition is the dangerous chemical PCP ("Angel Dust"). The results of using marijuana laced with addictives such as PCP are totally unpredictable and often lead to a violent person exhibiting bizarre thinking.

I emphasize once again that one of the really dangerous aspects of teenage and preteen marijuana use is that the user is much more susceptible to trying other drugs. This has been verified by a number of studies. Dr. Gabriel Nahas studied 5500 high-school students in New York who smoked marijuana frequently. Twenty-six percent began using harder drugs. Another study of 2200 heroin addicts at the U.S. Public Health Service Hospital in Lexington, Kentucky, showed that 74 percent began with marijuana.

This obviously does not mean that everyone who tries marijuana will become a heroin addict. What it does mean is that once the internal prohibition to avoid drugs has been overridden, then subsequent drug usage is highly likely if the opportunity to experiment is present. And the opportunity definitely *is* present everywhere—from grade schools through colleges, from blue-collar workers to top-level executives, from ghettos to Beverly Hills. All one needs to do to see the extent of drug usage is watch TV or read any newspaper or magazine.

A survey by the National Institute on Drug Abuse of teenagers and young adults showed a startling increase in use. In 1962, 1 percent of twelve- to seventeen-year-olds admitted using marijuana; in 1979, 31 percent admitted using marijuana (many professionals feel this figure is a very low estimate). In 1962, 4 percent of eighteen- to twenty-five-year-olds said they used marijuana, and by 1979 this figure rose to 68 percent! The tendency to use grass obviously has been increasing. Many teenagers—in fact, almost all the teenagers I see in my hospital program—complain of such great use of marijuana that they cannot avoid coming in contact with it daily, either at school or in the neighborhood.

Most of the benefits teenagers mention they derive from smoking marijuana revolve around the "high." This is a mild state of euphoria characterized by a feeling of well-being, gaiety, hilarity, and talkativeness. Early use often results in an increased awareness of color, sound, and taste. For these reasons concerts, movies, and eating sweets are favorite pastimes during a high.

Escape from boredom is another reason that is often cited. Obviously the more a kid uses marijuana to escape boredom, the less skills she is developing as she continues to grow. Chronic users often feel that the *only* way to deal with boredom is by smoking marijuana. Unfortunately, many people become chronic users in a very short time, often within months of their first experiments with marijuana.

I believe the subtle and most dangerous effect of marijuana is the gradual development of a psychological dependency on it. This is generally at the expense of developing effective coping skills. The use of the drug becomes *the* coping skill, and teenagers are especially prone to this. Once a pleasant feeling state is derived from marijuana, the adolescent often turns to marijuana to allay *any* anxiety.

Anxieties that are common during adolescence center around conflicts with parents, school, and friends. A convenient way to deal with these anxieties is to "tune out" by being stoned. All the problems are easily forgotten during the state of euphoria. Awareness of them returns once the high subsides, so the child has the choice of dealing with the anxieties or getting high again. He usually chooses the latter if he can.

Once marijuana no longer relieves the anxieties and conflicts (a common occurrence as anxieties accumulate), then a drug with stronger effects is often tried. I hope all parents will read that last sentence again, because it is very important. Of the nine thousand patients treated by our program over the years, at least 90 percent started their drug use with marijuana. Do not let your child continue smoking marijuana, or it may become the first of many drugs he uses during his life.

All the effects of marijuana I just mentioned also apply to hashish, hash oil, and THC. Marijuana is the weakest of the four drugs; so that the signs and symptoms of marijuana use are identical and exaggerated with the other three drugs.

HASHISH

Black Russian, blond hash, hash, kif

Hashish is a very potent substance that is also derived from the *Cannabis sativa* plant. It is much higher in THC content than marijuana and often eight to ten times as strong. Hashish is a resin of the Cannabis plant. It includes fibers that are bound together by various oils, and has the appearance of a rock or a piece of slate. Color varies from brown to black.

The usual method of ingesting hash is by smoking it in a pipe or sprinkling it on marijuana, although it can be eaten in various forms, such as cooked in brownies. Due to the increased amount of THC present, the high is more euphoric than with marijuana, lasts one to three hours, and is generally considered an increased marijuana high. There is heightened awareness of sensations such as taste, sight, and sound.

Hashish can also produce hallucinations, and in many people this leads to intense anxiety and paranoia. Some experience severe confusion and panic. "Bad trips"— frightening experiences while high—are much more frequent with hashish and hash oil than with marijuana.

There is much evidence that prolonged use leads to an enormous psychological dependence on the drug, just as it can with chronic use of marijuana. Although hashish is not as prevalent as marijuana in the United States, it is definitely available and used. Most of it is smuggled in from the Mideast.

HASH OIL

black oil, honey oil, Indian oil, oil, red oil, smash

Hash oil is two to four times as potent as hashish and as much as thirty times as potent as marijuana. It is a sticky liquid that varies in color from clear to black. This by-product of the Cannabis plant is produced by boiling the marijuana or hashish in a solvent, then filtering out the waste. The resulting liquid is extremely potent because it contains an enormously high percentage of THC.

Because of this large amount of THC, only a few drops can cause an intense high. It is often dropped on cigarettes or marijuana joints or simply spread on rolling paper. Commonly it is smoked in a special opium pipe. Overdose, which is easy to achieve because of its strength, can result in paranoia, delirium, and hallucinations. As with hashish, overdose is obviously a dangerous state, because a person's reactions are totally unpredictable during this period.

THC *(delta-9-tetrahydrocannabinol)*

THC, the most potent psychoactive ingredient in marijuana, hashish, and hash oil (see above), is frequently sold on the streets. The truth, however, is that most people who think they are purchasing THC are not buying THC at all. It is practically unavailable, and most persons taking T, as it is often called, are actually buying another drug. The other drug can be almost anything and is usually PCP, which is extremely dangerous. THC, if it really were available, would be too costly to buy. The expense of the process of refining THC from the Cannabis plant has essentially limited true THC to use in medical research. However, finding something else being sold as THC is hardly unusual, as there are few who will attest to the honesty of people who sell drugs for a profit.

ALCOHOL

booze, brew, (names of common mixed drinks), hooch, white lightning, suds, vino, moonshine, home-brew

Alcohol is the drug most often used in our country, and its use is on the increase in the teenage and young adult population. Much of the problem is that many people do not consider alcohol a drug. This is a dangerous misconception, to say the very least. I have interviewed thousands of parents who have condoned their children drinking alcohol just "as long as they don't smoke pot."

In many ways alcohol is more dangerous than marijuana, and it is definitely a mistake to consider either drug to be relatively benign or safe. Teenage alcoholism is a very real disease which often progresses into adult alcoholism. Recent estimates of deaths caused by alcohol place it as the third cause of death in the United States (after cancer and heart disease).

Many studies indicate that alcohol is responsible for about a fifth of the population in mental hospitals and about a third of suicides yearly. Although alcohol used in small amounts is not dangerous, the use of large amounts is very risky. In the teenage population it is even more of a problem, for most adolescents mix alcohol with other drugs. In many of these cases and in a number of ways, the combination is lethal. Alcohol mixed with depressants such as barbiturates can easily lead to an overdose situation, because the two drugs have a synergistic, or potentiating, effect on each other. Alcohol in combination with marijuana causes grosser distortions in time sense and judgment than either drug used singly. Studies showed that 17 percent of all fatal traffic accidents in one state were caused by the drivers' use of marijuana, and another 50 percent of drivers in deadly accidents had alcohol in their bloodstreams. That accounts for over 67 percent of the traffic deaths in that state.

Well over 250,000 people have been killed in traffic accidents caused by alcohol in the last decade. This figure does not include the millions who have been injured or the millions of families who have been destroyed by these tragedies. Because of this national horror, many states have become much tougher in dealing with drunk drivers. Fines are being increased, license suspensions are more frequent, and jail sentences are being imposed for first offenders.

Alcohol has become a very serious national health problem. Thousands of employers have felt it necessary to establish alcohol programs on the job or to find alcohol programs at nearby hospitals. The cost in lost productivity is estimated to be at least billions of dollars annually. Many companies estimate that each time they lose an employee, it may cost $40,000 or more to train a new person.

Alcohol is a drug that is easily attainable by adolescents, fairly inexpensive, and socially accepted in most circles. People drink not only to relieve tension but also to fit in, to present a sophisticated or "macho" image, and to celebrate certain occasions. When it is used for the wrong reasons, such as coping with frustration, a user will soon find that he develops tolerance of the effects of alcohol and must begin to increase his consumption to achieve the same desired effect. This is how alcohol addiction begins to develop. Any drug that has the characteristic of tolerance can become addicting, and alcohol is one of the most addicting of all drugs—it is physically addicting and it produces psychological dependence; that is, a person can feel that he must have a drink without actually going through withdrawal if he does not have one.

Alcohol is best classified as a depressant or a sedative-depressant. It acts on the central nervous system in many of the same ways that a barbiturate does. Once it is ingested, alcohol causes various responses. For some drinkers it feels like a stimulant, giving them increased energy. Others feel more of a tranquilized or sedated effect. It begins to act rapidly, and the effects are felt within a few minutes.

Ingesting a few ounces of hard liquor may cause a lessening of anxiety, impovement in self-confidence and esteem, and a general feeling of calm. Drinking over six ounces begins to cause some reversal of the euphoric mood, decline in self-confidence, unsteadiness, lack of concentration, and memory impairment. At this point speech is slurred, time and distance distortions appear, and behavior can become erratic, even violent.

Gross inebriation or intoxication occurs with a few more ounces. This is a sight we have probably all seen. It is characterized by loss of judgment, responsibility, equilibrium, memory, and thinking. The person is quite obviously drunk and may be very unpredictable.

Drinking more than this can cause a life-threatening situation. Coma and respiratory depression can lead to death. Among the real dangers of alcohol abuse, besides the possibility of developing alcoholism, are violent behavior, loss of reflexes and distortions leading to motor accidents, and bodily damage to the kidneys, brain, liver, and stomach. Vitamin deficiencies and peripheral nerve damage are also caused by alcohol.

Once a person has developed tolerance and then addiction, she may not safely cease her alcohol consumption. If she does, she may go through a most serious state—alcohol withdrawal. Withdrawal must occur in a hospital setting, because if a person develops delirium tremens (the DTs), she very well may die. Withdrawal symptoms include shakiness, tremors, anxiety, nausea, vomiting, diarrhea, cramps, hallucinations, convulsions, heart and circulatory failure, and coma, sometimes death. Withdrawal from alcohol is much more serious than withdrawal from heroin. The most similar drug withdrawal is from barbiturates.

In my view, alcohol is a very insidious, almost overlooked dangerous drug whose abuse the general population sees mainly as a problem in adults. This is far from an accurate picture. I have had to withdraw teenagers as young as fourteen from alcohol, and they exhibit the same symptoms as adults. Parents interested in preventing drug abuse in their children or adolescents must understand that alcohol is just as serious a problem as sleeping pills, pot, or heroin.

Many studies have shown that a greater number of alcoholics develop in families where one or both of the parents are alcoholics. In many cases the alcoholism can be traced back for generations. Some people feel it is heredity, but others of us feel that it is just as likely a learned experience. If a youngster grows up seeing the adults in his life use alcohol to deal with problems, he will feel that this is an acceptable way for him to handle frustration.

Teenagers tend to ignore warnings about drugs, especially if the drug is legal for older persons. This is compounded when the parents drink, even though they may drink moderately and without any apparent adverse effects. Much of the problem lies with a youngster not having the emotional maturity to drink responsibly (the same could be said for millions of adults, also). A youngster's psyche is not yet formed, and he does not have the coping skills to deal with many of the normal frustrations of everyday life, not to mention the tremendous pressures of just being an adolescent. If he uses any drug, including alcohol, and finds that it does relieve tension, it very often becomes his main coping device, as we've noted in reference to marijuana. This prevents the adolescent from developing newer, more effective means for dealing with disappointment and strife.

Since drinking is such an acceptable behavior for American adults, and since so many adults develop alcoholism, it is very important that adults examine their own drinking behavior to determine if their pattern is indicative of impending alcoholism. Adults should ask themselves to answer the following questions honestly:

1. Do you find yourself needing a drink for a little extra energy?
2. Does your drinking increase at all when you are under pressure?
3. Do you drink more than usual following an argument or a disappointment?
4. Have you ever had a "blackout" following which you could not remember some of the events that happened when you were drinking or could not remember coming home?
5. Do you drink more now than when you first started drinking?
6. Does it take more alcohol to feel relaxed than it used to?
7. Do you ever feel like you must have a drink? Do you feel uncomfortable if alcohol is not present?
8. Are you ever upset with yourself for drinking too much?
9. Do you ever tell yourself you need to drink less?
10. Do you avoid certain people when you are drinking, such as friends of your family?
11. Do you ever drink excessively for a long period, like one or two days?
12. Do people ever make comments about the amount or frequency of your drinking?
13. Are you more irritable than usual if you can't have a drink?
14. Do you have periods of lethargy or listlessness?
15. Do you have periods of depression?
16. Do you ever hide your drinking?
17. Do you drink alone?
18. Do old friends avoid you? Do you still get invited to parties?
19. Does your family mention your drinking? Do they say it is a problem or that it bothers them?
20. Is your health worse?
21. Do you eat less when drinking?
22. Do you ever think of suicide?
23. Do you ever have "visual hallucinations"—see things that are not there—while you are drinking or a few days after you stop drinking?
24. Do you ever have body tremors or shaking of your hands?
25. Have you ever had an accident or been stopped while driving and drinking?

This questionnaire is a guide for adults. It contains many situations that are present in early, middle, and even late stages of alcoholism. If you answered more than three questions yes, then I would advise you to try to stop drinking completely. If you are unable to stop, you have a definite alcohol problem.

Even if you do not feel you are an alcoholic, it is wise to assess what effect your drinking, if it is only "social" drinking, may be having on your child. If your teenager is abusing drugs, your drinking confirms that using an artificial chemical is acceptable. If the child is younger, he will also feel that his family accepts drinking—which it may—but the preteen may begin using alcohol much earlier than the parents would ever expect.

If a teenager is already having an alcohol problem, then a drug-abuse program such as a hospital treatment program, followed by a good twelve-step program such as AA offers (or other programs for teenage abusers), is an absolute necessity. The sooner treatment begins, and the more involved the total family, the better the chances for recovery.

DEPRESSANTS
barbiturates, methaqualone, nonbarbiturates, benzodiazepines, meprobamate

Depressants are highly abusable drugs that often produce a very severe withdrawal when their use is decreased or terminated. Taken as prescribed by a physician, they relieve anxiety, irritability, and tension and aid sleep. Higher doses can produce intoxication accompanied by a sense of well-being similar to alcoholic intoxication, depression, apathy, and impairment in speech, judgment, and control of motor functions.

Depressants include a number of different drugs that have a wide range of actions. They are all potentially addictive, although the benzodiazepines (Valium, Librium) are somewhat less so. The barbiturates, Doriden, and Quaaludes have the highest amount of addiction, but *all* these drugs produce a psychological dependency in people who are prone to depend on chemicals to solve their problems.

In the drug subculture, depressants are used for a variety of purposes. One reason is to get high. This is usually an attempt to allay anxiety and cause an alteration of consciousness simultaneously. Another purpose is to ease the pain of withdrawal from more addicting drugs such as heroin. A third purpose is to decrease the anxiety from "flashbacks" caused by using hallucinogens.

Tolerance is a factor with all these drugs. As your child increases his tolerance for depressants, he must increase his dosage to obtain the desired effect. Finally the margin between an intoxicating dose and a lethal dose becomes so small that overdose is the result. Furthermore, these drugs are particularly dangerous when they are mixed with other chemicals, alcohol being an excellent example. Many of the deaths of entertainment personalities have been the result of an accidental overdose caused by combining barbiturates and alcohol.

The results of a severe overdose with a depressant drug include symptoms of a cold, clammy skin, weak and rapid pulse, shallow respiration, low blood pressure, coma, and death.

Another serious side effect is the extremely severe withdrawal syndrome that results from the abrupt termination or reduction of depressant intake. A person who has been abusing "downers" should definitely be detoxified in a medical setting that has experience in this area, and not all hospitals do.

Initially a patient may improve when these drugs are stopped, but the withdrawal syndrome is soon to follow. It includes anxiety, motor restlessness, nausea and vomiting, cramps, sweating, shakiness, and an increased heart rate. Following this initial phase, a more severe syndrome that includes grand mal–like seizures ensues. A great number of those who suffer convulsions will then develop a delirium state similar to the delirium tremens (DTs) of alcohol withdrawal.

BARBITURATES

amies, barbs, blockbusters, bluebirds, blue devils, blue heavens, blues, candy, Christmas trees, downers, downs, goofballs, idiot pills, Mexican reds, nebbies, nemmies, nimbies, phennies, pink ladies, pinks, purple hearts, rainbows, redbirds, red devils, reds, sleepers, sleeping pills, tooies, yellow jackets, yellows

Barbiturates are prescribed for sleep and sedation, but a person who is abusing them obtains a stage of excitement prior to the sedative effects. Again, higher doses can lead to respiratory and cardiac failure, coma, and death.

These drugs were discovered in the seventeenth century but were not used heavily in America until the twentieth century. By the 1930s it was apparent that the effect produced by chronic use of barbiturates was similar to that of alcohol.

Barbiturates include a large number of drugs that are classified according to their length of action once they are in the body. Some of the brands most desirable to abusers are Tuinal, Seconal, Nembutal, and Amytal. They are short- to intermediate-acting, with an onset time of twenty to forty minutes and a duration of up to six hours. The shorter-acting ones have too brief a period of action to satisfy an abuser, and the longer-acting ones, with effects lasting eight to sixteen hours, are much too lengthy for most users.

Barbiturates, as well as the other depressants mentioned, have valid medical uses, including alleviation of tension, anticonvulsant properties, induction of sleep, sedation, and relief of minor pain. These drugs are relatively cheap by prescription, but their price increases on the street.

Usually the tablets or capsules are swallowed, but some

users inject them intravenously for a greater "rush" feeling. Injection is highly dangerous and can result in abscesses if an infection occurs as well as overdose from an enormous amount entering the circulatory system at once.

The effect of the barbiturate is to depress the nerve signals in the brain (therefore their classification as depressants). This then causes a depression of various physiological functions, such as a decrease in heart and respiration rates and a lowering of blood pressure. Higher doses progress the abuser from relief of anxiety to anethesia, coma, and death.

In the short term, barbiturates are similar to alcohol, causing a lessening of tension. Indifference arises, muscle tension is lessened, a feeling of mild euphoria may occur, and sleep eventually ensues. This is obviously a way to avoid dealing with any painful feelings or problems.

The long-term effects are more serious—constant fatigue, loss of memory and attention, instability, slurred speech, incoordination of gait, heightened anxiety, tremulousness, and poor judgment—and are all part of the picture of a chronic "barb" user. Other common effects are paranoia and violence.

METHAQUALONE *(Quaalude, Mandrax)*

ludes, sopers, 714s

This drug is one of the most commonly used among the teenage and young adult population. A nonbarbiturate that is a central nervous system depressant, it is produced under a number of different names; Quaalude, produced by Rorer, being the most common. The 150-milligram white pill reads "Rorer 712"; the 300-milligram white pill says "Rorer 714" on it.

Other brands include Sopor, Optimil, Somnafac, Parest, Biphetamine T, Thazole, and Mandrax (English). Mandrax is definitely a favorite of teenagers, but the terms *Quaalude* and *Mandrax* are often interchanged.

Methaqualone has a sleep-inducing quality because it reduces the nerve transmissions in the brain. An abuser gets high by fighting the induced sleep and staying awake to experience a state of incoordination, lessening of inhibitions, slight aphrodisia (for some), a feeling of lightness, and friendliness.

Tolerance can develop rapidly, and the amount of drug needed to overdose is only 2400 milligrams (eight 300-mg. tablets). Death by overdose is a very real possibility with this drug.

As with other drugs for which tolerance develops, a person can become both psychologically dependent on and physically addicted to methaqualone. The withdrawal symptoms include fatigue, tension, dizziness, dry mucous membranes, cramps, tremors, vomiting, and depression. A most serious withdrawal symptom is a withdrawal convulsion—a not uncommon occurrence in a Quaalude user who quits without medical supervision.

Furthermore, the combination of methaqualone with other drugs, such as alcohol, can produce a situation that is lethal. The drugs potentiate each other, causing greater depressant effects, thus leading quickly to respiratory arrest and death.

Another complication is overdose. Overdose on methaqualone is common, with symptoms that include convulsions, delirium, DTs, and hemorrhaging. This is a medical emergency that should be treated immediately by a qualified hospital. A person who has overdosed on methaqualone must be closely supervised; the same holds true for detoxification from methaqualone.

OTHER NONBARBITURATES

This group of sleeping pills includes Placidyl, Doriden, Noludar, and chloral hydrate. These drugs produce sleep, but their effectiveness wears off in a few weeks. Sleep is usually quick and lasts six to eight hours.

These drugs can be very habit forming. If one becomes addicted to one of them, as is frequent with Doriden, the withdrawal will be quite similar to that described for barbiturate withdrawal. I generally use an anticonvulsant and a barbiturate; I substitute the barbiturate for the nonbarbiturate by using a long-acting barbiturate, phenobarbital. Then I withdraw the patient gradually from phenobarbital.

Many deaths are attributable to these drugs by accidental or intentional overdose. They are very unsafe and should be removed from medicine cabinets if children or teenagers live with you.

BENZODIAZEPINES *(Valium, Librium, Tranxene, Ativan, Serax, Dalmane, Cloropin, Verstran)*

These drugs are marketed as minor tranquilizers, sedative-hypnotics, or anticonvulsants. They have no antipsychotic qualities and should not be confused with major tranquilizers such as Thorazine, Mellaril, Haldol, and Prolixin.

Prescribed in amounts that literally stagger the imagination, hundreds of millions of dollars' worth of Valium and Librium are sold yearly. They both have definite medical indications, such as relief of tension, reduction of muscle spasms, control of grand mal seizures, and as a preoperative sedative for surgery.

Some physicians and psychiatrists have overprescribed drugs in this category. If relief of anxietey is what the patient needs, Valium may seem to be the answer. What it does, of course, is diminish anxiety, but not the problem that is causing the anxiety. The person feels temporarily improved—and then the anxiety resumes. The impression most people have is that anxiety is the problem, but anxiety is the symptom—the problem that the person is struggling with consciously or unconsciously causes this symptom of anxiety.

Although these benzodiazepines have a greater margin

of safety than do the barbiturates, they can be—and are—abused drugs. The abuse occurs either by using more than the prescribed dose or using it in conjunction with other substances, such as alcohol. Benzodiazepines are potentiated by alcohol, barbiturates, and other drugs and are implicated in 10 percent of drug-abuse emergencies.

Benzodiazepines were initially abused by people who had been taking them by prescription from a doctor. As they continued to take them for months, then years, they became both psychologically dependent and physically addicted. Some effects of chronic usage include fatigue, tremors, confusion, drowsiness, diminution of sex drive, and severe depression. Psychotic reactions, rages, and an increase in excitability may also occur.

Withdrawal should be done in a hospital. The withdrawal syndrome usually begins seven to ten days after cessation of the drug. I have seen withdrawal symptoms of increased irritability and sleeplessness last for some months after Valium has been stopped.

More teenagers are using Valium and Librium, as well as other benzodiazepines, because of their easy accessibility in their parents' medicine cabinets. They are sold at school and in local hangouts and are frequently used in conjunction with other drugs by adolescents.

MEPROBAMATE *(Miltown, Equanil, Kesso-Bamate, SK-Bamate)*

Meprobamate was the first "minor" tranquilizer introduced to the public, becoming available in 1950. It does relieve anxiety, tension, and muscle spasms, but it does not cause sleep at clinical, or generally prescribed, levels. It is less toxic than the barbiturates, but tolerance, psychological dependence, and physical addiction definitely can occur. This drug is commonly found in medicine cabinets, as hundreds of tons of meprobamate are sold annually.

The withdrawal syndrome and overdose situation are similar to that of the barbiturates. The dose of meprobamate needed for death to occur is much higher than for barbiturates, but the combination with alcohol or other depressants increases the lethal effect.

This is a potentially dangerous drug to keep in a house with teenagers present. As there are a number of brand names for meprobamate, it might be best to check with your physician for information about *any* unknown drug in your medicine cabinet.

STIMULANTS
caffeine, amphetamines, cocaine

There are a variety of stimulants that kids use, some legal and some not. The two most common are caffeine and nicotine. I am going to emphasize caffeine, amphetamines, and cocaine in this section. I will refer the reader to the U.S. Government Printing Office for publications on nicotine.

Users of stimulants rely on these drugs to give them more energy, fight off fatigue, alleviate depression, and experience a "rush" or other state of euphoria. These drugs are frequently mixed with drugs having opposite effects, such as the depressants. Many people use stimulants to start out their day and a sleeping pill to aid sleep at night or to cut the edge off "coming down" from the stimulant.

CAFFEINE

Although I rarely treat a person for caffeine abuse alone, caffeine is a significantly dangerous and often abused drug. Small amounts of it are found in tea and coffee (100 mg. per cup), cola drinks, chocolate, and cocoa. Persons using caffeine in this form usually do not develop addiction, but I have seen cases of addiction to cola drinks in which people consume cola constantly throughout their waking hours.

The caffeine present in coffee or tea produces a slight increase in energy, pep, and concentration. Most persons are able to keep their consumption to a steady amount daily, say two to four cups of coffee. Some studies have shown that people who drink over five cups of coffee daily can suffer mild withdrawal symptoms if they stop their caffeine intake abruptly. This is usually felt as increased irritability, tiredness, and lethargy.

Young children often consume large amounts of caffeine. Since their bodies are small, a can of cola will actually be giving them more caffeine per pound of body weight than a cup of coffee provides for an adult. Add on a few chocolate bars to a number of cola drinks and you have a child who may be ingesting a few hundred milligrams of caffeine daily. He may be overly irritable and anxious and have difficulty sleeping.

A dangerous use of caffeine is now prevalent in our teenage population because of the explosion of the sale of "lookalike" stimulant drugs. Called lookalike as they are often exact replicas of amphetamines in their shape and color, these drugs usually contain large amounts of caffeine—300 to 500 milligrams per tablet, and occasionally much more. Sold by mail order through many magazines such as *High Times,* they are technically legal at this writing and are potentially lethal.

An average-size user will feel the effects of these pills within a few minutes. The initial feelings are increased energy, improved concentration, increased rate of the heart and pulse, elevation of blood pressure, secretion of stomach acids, and increased circulation. If the pill contains larger amounts of caffeine, symptoms of irritability, nervousness, insomnia, rapid heartbeat, gastrointestinal irritation, and diarrhea will follow.

As a user has no way of knowing how much caffeine he is ingesting or what else is present in the pill, overdose can occur. This situation results in confusion, disorientation, violence, bizarre thoughts and behavior, and convulsions. Death usually occurs at 10 grams (10,000 milligrams), and twelve deaths have recently been reported of caffeine overdose.

Withdrawal symptoms include agitation, shakes, lethargy, anxiety, and depression. It is more safely conducted in a hospital setting.

One of the problems with people taking these pills is that they may be taking a certain amount of these "fake speed" pills and then ingest real amphetamines without realizing the difference, as they look exactly alike. They also promote the use of illegal and more potent drugs in the future by creating a situation in which a youngster exhibits the same type of drug-using behavior as his peers who are using illegal drugs. This definitely increases his chances of moving into the use of illicit drugs.

The over-the-counter (nonprescription) diet suppressants can act in a similar way to caffeine pills and will probably be abused by a certain number of people when they cannot obtain amphetamines or other strong stimulants. In my opinion, they should be removed from the market, as their effectiveness in suppression of appetite seems to be short acting and their availability offers yet another drug to abuse.

AMPHETAMINES

A, beans, bennies, benzies, black beauties, black mollies, bombita, browns, coast-to-coasts, crank, cranks, crystal, crossroads, dexies, eye-openers, greenies, hearts, jelly beans, L.A. turnabouts, lidpoppers, meth, pep pills, skyrockets, speckled birds, speed, uppers, ups, wake-ups, whites

Amphetamines, known as speed or uppers in the drug culture, were first used medically in the late 1920s. By the early 1970s over thirty different preparations of amphetamines were available to the public. The first heavy use occurred during World War II, when both Allied and Axis troops were issued amphetamines to combat battle fatigue and increase the soldiers' endurance.

Following this period the drug was used to combat depression, improve concentration, and, paradoxically, treat hyperactivity in children. Eventually people who needed to stay awake for long hours, such as truck drivers and students, began to use uppers to stay awake. A black market of inexpensive amphetamines eventually began to supply the need and is flourishing today with more business than ever before.

Amphetamines can be categorized as stimulants, along with cocaine, caffeine, nicotine, phenmetrazine (Preludin), and methylphenidate (Ritalin). The main types of amphetamines are amphetamine, dextroamphetamine, and methamphetamine. These three types are very similar in their effects, and a lot of the difference seen in users is dependent on the amount used and the route of administration. All three create a long-acting cocainelike effect by stimulating the central nervous system.

The most common amphetamines are Benzedrine and Biphetamine, while the dextroamphetamines are represented by Dexedrine, Appetrol, and Synatran. A combination of dextroamphetamine and amobarbital is sold as Dexamyl. Other combinations with various drugs, such as methaqualone, are also available.

The most powerful group is the methamphetamines and includes Methedrine, Desoxyn, and Ambar. Other drugs, such as Preludin, Ritalin, and Tenuate, differ chemically from the true amphetamines but are considered here because their actions are so similar.

These drugs come in a variety of forms, including tablets and capsules. They are usually swallowed but can also be snorted or injected. The term "speed freak" refers to a person who abuses speed by injection to receive a "rush" feeling as the drug enters the bloodstream directly. This is the most serious form of abuse of amphetamines and can have disastrous effects. The term "speeding" means that someone is injecting himself repeatedly with amphetamines.

Because of our country's concern with appearing slim and healthy, many persons began to use these drugs to curb their appetite (an effect of the drug which is not usually long lasting). Because tolerance to this drug develops, a person using it had to increase the dosage or frequency constantly to continue to suppress his appetite. Lately doctors and health officials have decreased the amount of drugs prescribed, but the illegal market easily takes up the slack by making them readily available.

The drug works by stimulating the central nervous system. This causes the feeling of having more energy but also causes a racing of the heart, blood pressure, and pulse rate. It is quickly absorbed into the bloodstream even when it is ingested rather than injected. Users come to feel elated, confident, even omnipotent. They feel that they are functioning intellectually at a higher level, more productive, and full of energy. This state is soon followed by a more mellow euphoria, with a continuation of the heightened mood.

As the drug begins to wear off, in two to four hours, irritability, agitation, fatigue, and eventually a "let-down" depression start to set in. Frank paranoia is very commonly seen, and many persons begin to develop a paranoid delusional system, often centering around people trying to harm them or capture them and place them in jail. This "amphetamine psychosis" is extremely similar to a schizophrenic psychosis and is very dangerous both to the users and the people they come into contact with.

Many people tend to increase their use of the drug gradually and may continue to abuse it for days at a time. Loss of appetite and then loss of weight are common findings. Many users look much older than their age because their bodies have been functioning at an increased metabolic rate for a long time, and they have essentially aged rapidly. Other common findings are insomnia, formication (a feeling that bugs are under the skin), compulsive mannersisms such as foot tapping, and extreme agitation. All the effects of using a needle, such as ulceration, hepatitis, and liver damage, are also possible.

Overdose is serious and includes various chest and muscle pains and unconsciousness and can end in coma, convulsions, and paralysis. Tranquilizers are often effective in treating the overdose, and many users combine sedatives or depressants with their amphetamines to ease the "coming-down" period as the drug effect wears off.

Although there is disagreement as to whether amphetamines are physically addicting, there is little disagreement that they produce a high amount of psychological dependence. Withdrawal is not usually difficult but should be done in a hospital, under close supervision, and followed immediately by a drug-abuse treatment program. Many people show a decrease in intellectual capacity after prolonged use of these stimulants, and the possibility of brain damage exists.

A common denominator of amphetamine abusers is that they almost invariably feel depressed. Many of these people chose amphetamines because they temporarily alleviated their depression. Others may be depressed as a consequence of using the drug and experiencing the "letdown" depression that invariably follows. More teenagers are abusing amphetamines now than ever before, usually in conjunction with other drugs, particularly marijuana, alcohol, and depressants such as Quaaludes, even though laws are very strict and penalties great for the sale or possession of amphetamines.

COCAINE

big C, blow, burese, C, Carrie, Coke, Corine,
dream, dust, dynamite, flake, gold dust, heaven
dust, joy powder, lady, nose, nose powder, rock,
snow, snowbird, superblow, toot, white, white girl,
speedball (mixed with heroin)

Cocaine, the glamour drug of the seventies and very possibly the eighties, has been with us for centuries. What is this often-used drug taken by rock stars, praised in musical lyrics, worshiped by some of the wealthiest people in the country? What are its effects and its dangers?

Many people are now asking these questions as greater numbers of youths and "responsible" adults begin to obtain a new type of high and return again and again to cocaine.

Cocaine was originally used at least twelve hundred years ago by the Incas of Peru in the form of chewed coca leaves. The Inca ruler would dispense the leaves during religious ceremonies and as rewards for service. It was apparently considered a divine plant, and the coca leaves were the symbol of power and the fruitfulness of love. The ritual use of coca leaves permeated the ceremonial life of the Incas to the point that they buried the dead with pouches of coca leaves so that they would not be without it in the afterworld.

The Incas were conquered by the Spaniards in the mid-sixteenth century, and the first scientific report of coca use was made by Ponce de Léon in 1550. The Spaniards made attempts to suppress the chewing of coca leaves, assuming that the enhanced strength the Indians felt was actually a delusion of the devil. Eventually the Spaniards gave up suppression and began taxing the coca production—a 5 percent tariff on coca in 1795 yielded $2½ million.

Cocaine was then essentially ignored until the mid-nineteenth century, when it was isolated from coca in 1855 by Gardeke. The first well-known figure to investigate the drug was Dr. Sigmund Freud, well before he achieved fame as the founder of psychoanalysis. Between 1884 and 1887 Freud wrote five papers on coca and cocaine and suggested uses for it, such as a cure for morphine and alcohol addiction (which it isn't). Freud became disenchanted with cocaine in 1887, but a contemporary, Dr. Carl Koller, discovered the anesthetic properties of cocaine, and this led to acclaim by ophthalmologists who could use it in eye surgery. Physicians also used it as a "nerve block" for chronic pain.

The early heyday of cocaine use by the American population was from about 1890 to 1914. During this period many patent drugs and "soft drinks" contained cocaine. One familiar soft drink, Coca-Cola, was originally sold as a medicinal to cure "sick headaches, melancholy, etc.," and contained coca leaves, but in 1906 the formula was changed to include a decocainized coca leaf.

Due to federal legislation such as the Pure Food and Drug Act of 1906 and the Harrison Act of 1914, cocaine became illegal and was driven underground, its use occurring primarily in ghettos and among jazz musicians.

Cocaine began to regain its old popularity in the early 1970s, when smuggling cocaine became prominent since the amphetamines were assigned illegal status. As the country became more affluent, and as movies (such as *Easy Rider* and *Superfly,* both released in 1972), songs, and the mass media focused more on cocaine, a new subculture emerged. At least ten and a half tons are smuggled in annually, and the amount is probably much greater.

Where does it come from, how is it used, and what are the effects?

The coca plant is grown and harvested in Peru and Bolivia, but much of the cocaine is manufactured in Cuba and Chile. Essentially three processes must be completed before cocaine is sold to the consumer—first the cocaine is extracted from coca leaves, then it is mixed with hydrochloric acid, and finally it is diluted or "cut" with sugars such as mannitol, lactose, or inosital. Other ingredients are added to give it extra strength, so the buyer thinks he or she is receiving a higher quality of cocaine. Local anesthetics such as procaine or benzocaine are often used to enhance the quality, as well as stimulants such as caffeine or amphetamine.

Then it is smuggled by various routes into the United States, Miami, New York, and the Mexican border states being the three primary locations. It is marketed in a system similar to that which is used for heroin, but more rapidly, as it loses its potency with age. Since it is a white powder, it can be diluted easily, and this is how such enormous profits are made. Cocaine peddlers rarely provide more than 60 percent pure cocaine hydrochloride, and usually the amount is 5 to 40 percent. The remainder is "cut."

The usual method of using cocaine is by snorting—sniffing it through the nostrils, where it is quickly absorbed through the mucous membranes into the bloodstream. Other body orifices are also used occasionally, and a growing number of people are now injecting it directly into the bloodstream through their veins. This is the most dangerous method, since it causes people to become ever more dependent on it. "Running coke" (injecting cocaine) results in the heavy user shooting up twenty to thirty times daily. At $75 to $125 per gram (⅟₂₈ of an ounce), the cost is enormous and can run to hundreds of dollars daily. Many users have to resort to crimes such as burglary and robbery to support their habit. Some law enforcement officials feel that the high cost of drugs such as cocaine and heroin is a direct cause of the high crime rate.

The effects of the drug on humans consist of an increase of psychic energy, as it is a central nervous system stimulant; feelings of self-confidence, intense sexuality, excitability, anxiety, and euphoria. Most people who continue to use cocaine do so for a repetition of this state.

The physiological effects are increased heartbeat, pulse

and blood pressure; dilated pupils; nausea and vomiting; and occasionally hallucinations, impotence, insomnia, and confusion. A peculiar type of paranoid psychosis called formication is often seen (also called Magnan's Sign or cocaine bugs, it can be a symptom of amphetamine or alcohol abuse, too). This consists of the hallucination that insects or snakes are crawling on or under the skin, and the person often scratches his arms vigorously, to no avail. Another paranoid psychosis that is almost indistinguishable from acute paranoid schizophrenia may also develop.

Frequent use results in a number of dangerous conditions. Heavy sniffers usually destroy their mucous membranes, causing a continually runny nose and eventually a perforated nasal septum. Repeated doses can cause pallor, cold sweats, convulsions, fainting, toxic delirium, and respiratory failure and death. Unlike the effects of marijuana, there is very little doubt that death can result as a direct consequence of the pharmacological action of cocaine. This is usually preceded by respiratory depression and collapse of the cardiovascular system and often occurs when one injects a higher grade of cocaine than usual or a larger amount. Death also occurs among sniffers and may be related to the additives as well as the cocaine.

Given the horrible consequences of cocaine use, why do so many people begin and then continue to use this drug? My impression from treating adolescents who use cocaine is that a variety of situations occurs: many if not most have absolutely no idea of these side effects; some are polydrug users who are looking for a new thrill; and many are relatively affluent kids who have become bored with marijuana and are introduced to the drug in a familiar social setting, such as a cocktail party.

Little popular literature is available on the serious aspects of this dangerous chemical, and it is often viewed as being as innocuous as alcohol—which is also potentially dangerous.

The initial use usually involves sniffing cocaine low in

purity and strength, which causes some temporary euphoria, giddiness, and excitement. It is through repeated use
that people gradually develop the problems. There is disagreement as to cocaine's addictive qualities; many people
feel that since physical withdrawal symptoms are not common, as they are with heroin use, dependency is not a
problem. They ignore the fact that cocaine produces a psychological dependency that is surpassed by few chemicals.

Cocaine users are notorious for developing tolerance to
its effects and then increasing their usage and ultimately
"craving" cocaine. Depression often follows the euphoria,
and the tendency is strong to sniff or shoot more cocaine to
return to the euphoric state. This is essentially the same
vicious cycle that is seen in most forms of drug abuse,
dependence, and addiction.

In recent years many prominent figures in sports, entertainment, and other areas of public life have been associated with the use of cocaine. This has an enormous impact
on adolescents, who rationalize that since it is acceptable in
their idols, it is therefore harmless. They often use it to
identify with those same idols who hold so much signifi-
cance for them.

The most effective means of changing attitudes is through
the media, community awareness, and the schools. Government suffers from lack of credibility in the view of most
adolescents as well as many adults. Medical professionals
are lax in informing the public and usually lack knowledge
about specific "street drugs" unless they are directly involved in drug-abuse treatment. In many cases teenagers
are much more informed about the supposedly beneficial
effects of drugs, as they have used them lightly or heard
their peers speak only positively about them.

Prevention and treatment are essentially left to parents,
concerned citizens, and a handful of specialists in this area.
The number of cocaine-using youngsters treated by me
during the last three years has risen enormously, and it is

not uncommon to see young teens using cocaine, usually in combination with other equally dangerous drugs. If this is a sign of our times, it is time that parents, citizens, local government, and medical professionals band together to be heard in unison. We have joined to eradicate such illnesses as polio and smallpox—why not drug abuse?

HALLUCINOGENS/PSYCHEDELICS
(LSD, Psilocybin, Mescaline, PCP)

LSD, PCP, psilocybin, and mescaline are known to produce hallucinations in the user. Needless to say, many other drugs exist that also can produce hallucinations. Some of these, such as alcohol and hashish, are covered in separate sections. Other infrequently used drugs are not within the scope of this book, as I am attempting to present those drugs that are used commonly enough in our society to present a potential danger to our children.

Chemicals that distort objective reality are termed "hallucinogens." Their action on the body is one of exciting the central nervous system, and this causes alterations of mood from euphoria to severe depression. Severe distortions of time, sense, direction, and judgment ensue. In moderately large doses, delusions and hallucinations occur.

LSD (lysergic acid diethylamide)

acid, beast, Big D, blotter, blue acid, blue mist, California sunshine, coffee, cubes, cupcakes, domes, dots, haze, heavenly blue, Lucy in the Sky with Diamonds, mellow yellows, microdots, orange mushrooms, orange sunshine, paper acid, purple haze, purple microdot, strawberry fields, sugar lump, sunshine, 25, wedges, white lightning, window pane, yellows, zen

LSD, or "acid," is one of the most potent drugs known to humans. The dosage needed to produce a "trip," or intoxication, is extremely small. To give you an idea of the potency, heroin and cocaine are measured in grams, one gram being a common amount for an injection of heroin. LSD, on the other hand, is measured in micrograms, one microgram being equivalent to one-millionth of a gram. As little as 50 micrograms can produce a trip, and street dosages can contain 5000 micrograms or more. The amount of LSD in a tablet the size of an aspirin would cause a trip for about three thousand people.

LSD was originally discovered in 1938, and its effects became known in 1943. Dr. Albert Hofmann had been working on the twenty-fifth compound of a series of drugs related to lysergic acid, and he named this one LSD-25.

LSD has been researched in various areas since that first experience of Dr. Hofmann. The best-known proponent of LSD in America was Dr. Timothy Leary. Perhaps because of the great publicity given to LSD during the sixties, its use became widespread. The use of LSD eventually spread beyond the "hippies" or "flower children" of the 1960s to professionals as well as college, high school, and middle school students. It was popularized in a song by the Beatles called "Lucy in the Sky with Diamonds."

Prior to that time LSD was researched by various scientists. The US Army attempted to establish its effectiveness for brainwashing and for making prisoners communicate more freely. Initially some psychiatrists took LSD, believing that inducing a psychotic experience in themselves would better enable them to understand their psychotic patients. During the 1950s LSD in small doses was used with a variety of psychiatric patients. The initial impression was that LSD would loosen a person's internal inhibitions, thus allowing him to verbalize more freely. Depressed states, alcoholism, and terminal states of cancer were some of the situations in which LSD experiments took place.

Gradually the therapeutic uses of LSD were discontinued because a number of undesirable effects and hazards were found. Until the early 1960s LSD was supplied by

Sandoz Laboratories. When the Federal Drug Administration passed new laws regulating drugs because of the thalidomide tragedy, Sandoz began to restrict the distribution of LSD. This promptly resulted in an increase in the amount of LSD, as the formula was available from the US Patent Office and easy to synthesize. Illegal labs sprang up around the country, and by 1970 it was estimated that one- to two-million people had used LSD. This number increased to 15,800,000 persons by 1979, according to a National Institute on Drug Abuse survey.

A colorless liquid, LSD can be used in various forms. Initially it was often placed on sugar cubes. LSD was and still is inexpensive. The cost of a dose large enough for a trip ranges from $1 to $10.

Part of the reason for the popularity of LSD was the government's initial scare tactics about marijuana and confusing information about LSD. As mentioned earlier, the marijuana of the 1960s was of very low potency, containing usually 0.5 percent THC. As people experimented with this weak marijuana, they began to disbelieve government statements about marijuana and, by extension, any other drugs.

This was an unfortunate circumstance, as many drugs, particularly LSD, can cause serious problems. Then, to compound the problem, once the weak marijuana became acceptable to greater numbers of people, a higher-potency marijuana was developed that does have many of the effects the government publicized fifteen years ago.

LSD is generally considered harmful because of some serious side effects. Proponents of LSD feel that the "mind-expansion" potentials of the drug are its greatest attribute. In general, the course of an LSD experience is as follows. A person who ingests LSD usually experiences some anxiety and nausea; an increase in metabolic functions such as pulse rate, blood pressure, and heartbeat; a flushed face; and restlessness. The next phase is the "trip."

This state may be euphoric or extremely frightening, and usually lasts eight to twelve hours. Much of what happens at this point is dependent on the psychological state of the user, the setting he or she is in, the dosage of LSD, and the impurities present in it.

A pleasant trip is described as one in which all the senses are heightened and often merged. Colors take on new intensity, patterns take on dimensions, and smell and hearing are intensified. A loss of sense of time and body often occurs. Trivial incidents take on exaggerated meaning. Some people claim a heightened self-awareness and an experience of increased consciousness.

A bad trip is a very frightening experience. LSD is a "psychomimetic" drug—a drug that produces a state that mimics a psychosis. This includes frightening hallucinations (seeing or hearing things that do not exist), illusions (misperceptions of real events), and frank, overwhelming paranoid feelings and panic. Chronic anxiety states, decreased concentration, severe depression, suicide, homicide, aggression, bizarre behavior, and personality changes can occur.

The most severe reactions to LSD are panic, flashbacks, and psychosis. The panic state is one in which the user feels helpless and fears going crazy. A flashback is a recurrence of an LSD state long after the LSD has worn off, in which visual and auditory hallucinations may occur. The exact reason why this occurs is unknown, but one theory is that LSD is stored in fat cells and is occasionally excreted back into the bloodstream. This may occur at any time and is more likely when the person is under stress. Other theories dispute this idea.

An extended psychosis can develop, also. This may be a schizophreniclike state or a state of continuous hallucinations. The psychotic state may be of short duration (an acute psychosis) or may become chronic with prolonged use of LSD or other hallucinogens.

The full extent of the danger of LSD remains unknown,

since research was eventually curtailed. Some evidence exists that it can cause chromosome abnormalities, and it is certainly a dangerous drug to take during pregnancy as well as at any other time.

It probably could have been a useful therapeutic drug if it had been used only in controlled settings in small dosages (25 micrograms), given to people with very stable personalities.

Much of the problem now is the strength of the usual dose (5000+ micrograms), which is two hundred times as strong as the clinical dose. In addition, LSD may be synthesized incorrectly or have other substances added to it (adulteration). These substances are often phencyclidine (PCP) or amphetamines, which add to the possibility of a bad trip.

There is, unfortunately, no method to predict who will have a bad trip. For some people it happens the first time they try LSD; for others it does not occur until many experiments with LSD have taken place. Many persons, particularly those with unstable personalities or unformed psyches, which are common during the teenage years, develop a psychosis. This psychosis is often irreversible and may leave the person in a chronic paranoid psychotic state.

PSILOCYBIN *("Magic Mushrooms")*

magic mushroom, mushroom, los niños ("the children")

Psilocybin is a hallucinogen found in about 20 varieties of mushrooms. There are over 35,000 varieties of mushrooms in the world, so the chances of mistaken identification are great. Many types of mushrooms are poisonous, and few people are well versed enough to know which ones are safe. The use of these hallucinogenic mushrooms dates back thousands of years, to Central American Indians of that time.

Psilocybin can also be produced synthetically, but this is

an expensive procedure, and very little synthetic psilocybin is available on the streets. When it is produced, it is sold as tablets, capsules, or liquid. Most samples sold to the buyer are a combination of psilocybin, LSD, and PCP.

The potency of a psychedelic mushroom is enhanced by extracting the psilocybin, which is done by grinding the mushroom and soaking it in methyl alcohol. The residue is very potent. Psilocybin, like LSD, is usually ingested. Both drugs can be taken intravenously; the trip begins sooner with this route of administration.

Dr. Albert Hofmann, the scientist who discovered LSD-25, was the person who first isolated psilocybin from the mushroom *Psilocybe Mexicana Heim*. A second alkaloid, psilocin, was also isolated. It is equally as powerful. Once the mushroom is ingested, psilocybin, which is an unstable compound, is converted to psilocin. Psilocin appears to be the active substance that causes the medical and psychiatric effects of the mushrooms.

Psilocybin effects are similar to LSD effects but are of a shorter duration, usually lasting two to six hours. LSD is 150 to 200 times as potent as psilocybin, but equivalent doses produce a trip that is indistinguishable by the user.

The physical effects include dilation of the pupils; blurred vision; dizziness; muscular relaxation; decreased concentration; increase in pulse rate, blood pressure, and temperature; nausea; and anxiety. The trip begins forty-five to sixty minutes after ingestion and is characterized by visual and auditory hallucinations, isolation from the external world, disorientation, and giggling.

The most prominent effect is the change in visual sensation. This is described as a heightened awareness of colors, seeing new patterns of colors and objects, and a sharpness of definition of colors and objects. The user begins to become indifferent to the world, and the dreamlike state becomes his reality. He loses a sense of time and enters a world entirely of his own.

The dissatisfying or bad trip can include paranoid reactions, extreme anxiety that often leads to a panic state, disorientation, and depression. This may continue until the effect of the drug wears off or longer.

Users of both LSD and psilocybin develop tolerance to the drug, so that increased amounts must be taken to achieve the same trip. There is evidence that users of both drugs develop a cross-tolerance, so that more of either drug is needed for a trip. Tolerance to LSD and mescaline (see following discussion) can take less time to develop than does tolerance to psilocybin.

MESCALINE *(Peyote)*

beans, buttons, cactus, mescal, mescal buttons, moons, plants

A plant that grows in northern Mexico, the peyote cactus has been used by Indians there for centuries as part of their religious rites. Its use gradually spread to American Indian tribes, and members of the Native American Church of North America are exempt from United States laws governing the use of peyote.

Peyote is a small, spineless cactus that contains crowns. The crowns are cut off, dried, and eaten. Vomiting occurs in almost every case. After two hours of nausea, vomiting, pupillary dilation, and increased heart rate and blood pressure, the trip begins.

The initial stage may include increased sensitivity and visual hallucinations of extremely bright colors and designs. Indians tend to meditate during this period and are often vague in their description of the trip. They often see "visions" as part of the religious experience that is occurring.

The "hallucinations" are more properly described as "illusions," as it is usually an intensification and distortion of the real world that is being experienced. True hallucinations with this drug are uncommon. Increased sensitivity to sound is also present.

Other effects are anxiety, impairment of intellect, and exacerbation of underlying psychiatric problems (especially among psychotic users).

The most active drug causing the change is mescaline, an alkaloid found in the peyote cactus. However, other substances found in peyote are responsible for the trip also, as manufactured mescaline taken alone does not produce the same trip for the user. A dose of mescaline can last for twelve hours and also produces the hallucinogenic or illusionary features.

Its use by Indians has spread over the years, both for religious experiences and to relieve fatigue. Medicinal qualities are ascribed to the peyote by the Indians, but this is questionable.

Mescaline and peyote were abused by non-Indians more during the 1960s, but some usage still occurs. Because of the unpleasant effects of nausea and vomiting, most hallucinogenic users prefer LSD over mescaline.

Mescaline, like LSD and psilocybin, also produces tolerance, necessitating increased dosages for frequent users. The abuse potential is high for all three drugs.

PCP *(Phencyclidine)*

angel dust, animal tranquilizer, crystal, DOA dust, elephant tranquilizer, goon, horse tranquilizer, killer weed, mist, peace pill, sheets, supergrass, superweed, weed

Casual users of drugs have increased at an astounding rate during the last decade, and many have unknowingly taken a trip they were not expecting, often with disastrous effects.

PCP (phencyclidine) first appeared in the drug world in 1967. It was originally "discovered" in 1957 by researchers at Parke, Davis & Co., when its anesthetic effect on animals was observed by them. Investigations of its potent analgesic and anesthetic effects were discontinued in 1965 because of its severe behavioral effects on humans.

Starting in the early 1970s, many startling effects of the drug were described, including long-term psychotic episodes (breaks with reality). In spite of the obvious unpredictability and dangerous consequences of using PCP, its popularity spread like an epidemic, perhaps because of its availability and low cost.

Parents, teachers, legal system personnel, and professionals in drug abuse are faced daily with the problems that PCP causes. Because of its prevalence in the drug world, an understanding of its effects is important.

PCP is a white powder that dissolves in water. In its street form, however, it may appear as a liquid, tablet, or powder and is difficult for the user to recognize. It is *very often* misrepresented as being other drugs, and the inexperienced or unwary user often takes PCP without being aware of it.

In addition to being added to other drugs, often including marijuana, LSD, mescaline, amphetamines, opiates (such as heroin), cocaine, and barbiturates, PCP may contain many impurities, such as potassium cyanide. It is easily produced in a laboratory, and the chemicals used to make it are available because of widespread industrial use. To further complicate the situation, a number of drugs similar to PCP are being synthesized and can produce similar psychiatric symptoms. Some of these drugs are PCC, PCE, PHP, TCP, and ketamine.

The purity of the PCP is another problem. When it is sold as a powder ("angel dust") it is usually relatively pure (50–100% PCP). When it is sold in other forms, however, it often shows less purity (usually 5–35% PCP). The remaining 65 to 95 percent is often other dangerous contaminants.

The effects of using PCP can be altered slightly by the

route of ingestion. PCP was originally taken orally, but the user has little control over the amount that will be absorbed into the bloodstream. The more popular method currently is to smoke or inhale (snort) PCP, as that way the user can better determine the amount in her body and supposedly diminish the possibility of an overdose.

What are the specific effects of PCP, and its dangers? Why do so many people abuse this unpredictable chemical?

Most users report both positive and negative side effects, and those who continue to use the drug are usually trying to recapture the original positive experience. They are generally aware that negative effects are present (88% knew in one study). There is no reason to believe that a repeat experience will have the same result as the original experience, due to such variables as purity, types of adulteration chemicals, and route and amount of ingested PCP.

The positive effects noted have been increased sensitivity to stimuli, mood elevation, stimulation, inebriation, and dissociation. Euphoria is reported in only 8 percent of users. The effects that are unpleasant to the user include perceptual disturbances, restlessness, disorientation, anxiety, paranoia, irritability, hyperexcitability, mental confusion, speech difficulties, violence, bizarre behavior, auditory and visual hallucinations, feelings of impending doom and death, catatonic staring, generalized anesthesia and rigidity, long-term psychosis, convulsions, respiratory depression, coma, and death. Typical descriptions by users include the following positive effects: fantastic, "mind blowing," "super-high," "light," mellow, calm. However, the majority of those questioned gave negative responses of feeling rowdy, violent, numb, paranoid, isolated, unable to communicate, spacey, robotlike, uncoordinated, exhausted, depressed, lonely, bored, and insecure.

Psychosis can develop three to four days after PCP has been used and may occur after a single dose. The PCP psychosis is considered a psychiatric emergency, as the person is dangerous to himself and others because of depression, suicidal impulses, paranoia, and tendency toward violence. It must be treated immediately by a clinician who is skilled in this area.

PCP overdose occurs frequently and is life threatening. PCP remains in the urine for several days and should be tested for in all suspicious cases, as many people do not realize that they have taken PCP. Many persons with an overdose are misdiagnosed as having an acute psychosis, such as a schizophrenic breakdown.

So why the paradox of increased use of a drug that has a reputation for causing such severe reactions? This may be because the abuser feels he can avoid overdose by smoking or snorting the drug, or desires to repeat an initial good experience with PCP, or because of its increased availability, the desire to get high no matter what the consequences, peer pressure, or abusing PCP as an unknown addition to another street drug. Another reason is that for many people being high or stoned is the only mechanism they have developed to cope with feelings of anxiety, stress, boredom, or even life in general. In what I believe is a psychological dependency on the drug, they may feel trapped by it, but are unable to cease using it.

There is some question about its addictive properties, as monkeys will self-administer PCP when given the opportunity, but they will not administer other hallucination-producing drugs. Although it is not as physically addictive as such drugs as heroin or morphine, it does appear to create a high degree of psychological dependency, which I feel is the main problem to be dealt with in treatment. New skills must be learned to deal with all types of stress that one encounters, and the user must receive positive validation of his new coping devices for some time or a relapse is likely. Removal of the person from the negative peer group—his acquaintances who use drugs (usually 95% in

PCP studies)—is an important ingredient for successful treatment. Hospitalization is often necessary, as it separates the user from his group, decreases the possibility of continued use of PCP during recovery, and provides in-depth therapy, drug-abuse counseling, and contact with an aftercare drug-abuse program.

PCP is another dangerous chemical that our children and adolescents are exposed to frequently; it can cause fatal tragedies in a family with only one-time use. I feel parents can have excellent results in preventing PCP use by providing early education for their children, stressing the importance of drug education in schools, and organizing parent-awareness groups to disseminate this type of information to their communities. The more influential parents are in preventing all types of drug abuse, the less are the chances their own children will become victims of the drug world.

In 1978 over two hundred deaths and ten thousand emergency-room visits were attributed to PCP. The figures are probably much higher, as PCP is often sold as other drugs, especially THC (marijuana's active ingredient—a drug rarely found on the streets). Estimates from NIDA (National Institute on Drug Abuse) indicate that over 5½ million people have used it.

Because of the severe effects of PCP, in 1978 Congress passed legislation imposing stiff penalties for its manufacture or possession with intent to distribute. A first offense can carry a penalty of ten years of imprisonment and/or a $25,000 fine. A second offense can result in twenty years in prison and/or a $50,000 fine.

INHALANTS

gunk, gas, glue

The practice of inhaling substances to cause a euphoric state dates back many centuries. A relatively new phenomenon, however, is the widespread use among male juveniles (average age of 14).

In the last few years inhalants have begun to be used more frequently by the Anglo population also. It is a type of abuse that is difficult to identify and treat. Part of the problem lies in the legal, cheap availability of the products that are inhaled. Many studies indicate that inhalant abusers, or "huffers" as they are often known, are frequently loners who have severe psychological problems that they are attempting to avoid by inhaling; they often have a disruptive family life.

This description is often true of the chronic user, and about one-fifth of the people who experiment with inhalants progress to chronic usage. Many kids use inhalants as just another drug to experiment with, but others select it as their drug of choice, and they are the ones who exhibit chronic dependency on inhalants.

Inhalants comprise a number of substances, including anesthetics such as ether, chloroform, and nitrous oxide as well as many products found in the home and in retail stores.

The typical huffer tends to use substances such as aerosol cans that contain fluorinated or chlorinated hydrocarbons as a propellant for the product. The list includes spray deodorants, medications, polishes, paint, cleaners, sanitizers, and insecticides. Others include varnish, lighter fluid, nail polish and remover, gasoline, hair spray, spot remover, and spray-on cooking lubricants (like PAM). This is only a partial list, and a check under your sink or in your utility room will reveal more products, all of which are legal, inexpensive, and easy for a teenager to obtain.

Usage includes methods such as pouring the substance on a rag or spraying it into a small bag or balloon and sniffing it. Others inhale it through the mouth. Some people only use an inhalant once as an experiment, but chronic users may be high essentially all the time. Some people inhale in groups, but most frequently it is done alone.

Inhalation produces depression of the nervous system, lowering of inhibitions, and a state of delirium. There is gross impairment of thinking capabilities; confusion; slurred speech; incoordination; and a drunken, euphoric state. The person is attempting to produce a state of euphoria or elation, and once this is achieved, a dangerous situation develops because the person is so uninhibited that he often becomes violent and destructive. Hallucinations, illusions, and delusions are also common.

Physical distortions of weightlessness, floating, and numbness are common as the drugs act on the brain. Disorientation and distortion are quite common, and people lose control of their emotions also. Finally a state of drowsiness or sleepiness ensues, and the person may fall asleep.

Physical alterations include increase in heart rate, decrease in respiration, nausea, vomiting, diarrhea, pupillary dilation and changes in vision, cough, decreased appetite, unsteadiness, and rash.

Psychological dependence can develop rapidly, causing the user to inhale more fumes more frequently. As the psychological dependence develops, tolerance also increases, so the person enters a vicious cycle of escalating usage. Although physical addiction is questionable, many people report a number of withdrawal-like signs such as increased irritability, anxiety, and aggressiveness.

Although the effects of long-term use are not fully understood, there is no disagreement that inhalants pose a number of threats. These include cardiac arrest, cardiac rhythm abnormalities, and depression of the respiratory system with resultant cessation of breathing, loss of oxygen, and death. Another cause of death is from vaporizing the airway and preventing oxygen from being absorbed. Also found are liver damage, lead poisoning (often fatal), kidney damage, and changes in the structure of white and red blood cells.

As far as treatment is concerned, the inhaler is a special case with poor prognosis. Many drug-abuse programs have difficulty attracting these users to come for help, since they are often isolated individuals with little conscious need for social interaction and do not desire to change this situation. Specialized programs dealing only with inhalers are occasionally established. Intensive individual, group, and family therapy are often needed for success.

NARCOTICS
(Opium, Heroin, Methadone)

OPIUM, MORPHINE, DILAUDID, DEMEROL

Demerol: junk, stuff, white stuff
Dilaudid: Big D, D, junk, shit, stuff, white, stuff
Morphine: cube, dope, hard stuff, junk, morphie,
mud, sister, stuff, white stuff

The opium poppy, *Papaver somniferum*, has been available for thousands of years. Untold millions of persons have become addicted to it or its derivatives: morphine, heroin, and codeine. Synthetic narcotics such as methadone, Demerol, and Percodan are also highly addictive.

Opium is the natural product of the opium poppy, and morphine is the main addicting ingredient present in it. It was a legal drug in America until 1914 and was sold in grocery stores, by mail order, and in patent medicines, and was dispensed by doctors. Opium and its derivatives are now illegal, and synthetic narcotics are legal only by prescription. Penalties for illegal possession are quite stiff.

Opium comes in a bitter, sticky bar or is available in powder. Its fumes are usually inhaled by the user, although it can be eaten also. It produces a euphoric state that is filled with fantasy, apathy, and detachment. Many researchers feel that the user does not achieve any real pleasure from the drug but instead feels relief at the disappearance of awareness of frustrations and anxieties.

Morphine (morphine sulfate) is a drug that is an excellent painkiller but is highly addictive. It can be found in powder or liquid form, thus allowing it to be injected. This route of administration causes addiction much more rapidly than taking it orally. The initial pleasant effects of morphine are similar to opium, as morphine is responsible for the effects of opium.

Eventually users will become addicted to the drug if they continue to use it frequently enough. Unfortunately there is no way to predict at what point a user will become addicted. Once addiction occurs, the person must continue to use opium or morphine to avoid the pain of withdrawal. He will continue to need larger doses to remain in a "normal" state, so the possibility of overdose then becomes a factor.

Someone who becomes addicted to either drug begins to dread the withdrawal phase and will continually take the drug to avoid the chills, nausea, vomiting, aches, sweating, tremulousness, and anxiety that characterize withdrawal. Withdrawal should take place in a hospital setting, as it is complicated at times.

Certain drugs taken along with morphine or opium, such as alcohol or barbiturates, can prove disastrous and result in death for some individuals.

Morphine has been extensively researched by scientists and found to cause EEG changes, central nervous system depression (and occasionally stimulation), sedation, lethargy, confusion, exhaustion, nausea, vomiting, constipation, and increased blood sugar.

A very potent semisynthetic derivative of morphine, Dilaudid, has recently become a heavily abused drug. Although it can be ingested to get a high, most of the users I have treated have injected it intravenously. It is stronger than morphine, has fewer side effects, and is very addicting. The withdrawal is more painful than with heroin and takes five to seven days to complete in a hospital situation.

Quite a bit of Dilaudid seems to be available on the streets at this point, and a large black market is developing.

Another potent analgesic, Demerol, is also highly addicting if it is taken long enough. Used medically in a hospital for a short duration following surgery, it is usually not addicting. It produces euphoria and clouds the sensorium to some degree. Many persons with illnesses that produce chronic pain, such as severe backaches and migraines, become addicted to it. The other group that is prone to addiction is the medical profession, as its members have easier access to this drug than the general population.

HEROIN

big H, boy, brother, brown, brown sugar, crap,
doojee, dope, goods, H, hard stuff, Harry, horse,
joy powder, junk, ka-ka, poison, shit, smack,
smeck, snow, stuff, sugar, thing, white stuff

Heroin is the narcotic of choice of American users, partially because of its availability. Other countries have had more problems with opium, China being a good example.

Although the history of opiate derivatives being abused in America dates back to at least 1850, heroin gradually emerged as the opiate drug most frequently used. Until the 1960s it was predominantly found in minority groups.

An explosion in heroin usage has taken place since that time, and heroin has moved out of the ghettos and into middle-class America. By 1974 the estimate of heroin addicts reached almost 800,000 persons. By 1979 the National Institute on Drug Abuse estimated that 2,600,000 persons had tried heroin but had no accurate figures on the amount who were currently addicted.

The government has attempted various programs to limit the supply of heroin that is smuggled into America. At one point Turkish farmers were paid not to grow the poppy flower, and programs with Mexico have been tried with some success.

The Golden Crescent area, consisting of Iran, Afghanistan, and Pakistan, had an enormous crop in 1980 estimated at sixteen hundred metric tons, with the majority destined to go to America. Drug-enforcement agencies feel this is definitely increasing the heroin-addict population in America for a number of reasons.

First, there is now increased availability, with a concomitant drop in the cost of heroin. Second, the heroin is of a stronger potency than most previous supplies from Mexico and Turkey. Third, since cocaine is relatively expensive, many persons who use cocaine will switch to heroin to diminish their expenses. Unfortunately, the new heroin is so powerfully addicting that many former cocaine users will become heroin addicts.

Heroin is made by converting morphine in a laboratory. Heroin is more potent and more addicting than morphine. A person can become addicted in a matter of days to weeks, depending on the potency of the heroin and the frequency of usage.

As with opium and morphine, tolerance and physical addiction go hand in hand. As it takes more of the drug to achieve the same effect, the person becomes physically addicted and will experience withdrawal symptoms if the heroin is discontinued.

Heroin users generally prefer injecting the drug into their veins, although inhaling or smoking heroin occasionally occurs. Injection is, of course, the quickest way to become addicted. Initially an injection causes nausea in the experimenter, but past this phase a pleasant, euphoric state occurs. As the user tries to achieve this state over and over again, his tolerance is increasing, and he becomes addicted.

From the point of addiction on, the person then uses heroin to avoid the withdrawal symptoms. As he continues to "shoot" or inject heroin, he can remove himself from reality for periods of time, but it becomes necessary for him to inject himself more and more frequently to avoid withdrawal. As he begins to sweat, itch, and have chills and aches, he again must shoot up to avoid more severe withdrawal.

If he is unable to continue injecting heroin, he will enter the full withdrawal syndrome, which is characterized by sweating, chills, aches, cramps, diarrhea, sleeplessness, shaking, weakness, pain, and occasionally convulsions. Detoxification (withdrawal) should take place in a hospital setting rather than going "cold turkey" on the streets. Many of the symptoms can be lessened or alleviated by an appropriate withdrawal regimen administered by a physician.

Heroin produces many other complications besides addiction and withdrawal. Many law-enforcement agencies cite heroin addiction (and other drug abuses) as a chief cause of crime. With heroin costing from $50 to over $500 daily for an addict, stealing becomes a necessary means of supporting the habit. Since the person can hardly function at a steady job and his usage is constantly increasing, illegal means of obtaining money for the heroin must be resorted to.

The use of unclean needles for injection often causes hepatitis (serum or infectious), blood poisoning, and abscesses. Infection can occur in the lining of the heart (subacute bacterial endocarditis) and prove fatal.

Overdose is a common cause of death among heroin users. This can occur because of differences in potency in drug samples, adulterants in the heroin, or of other drugs in addition to heroin, leading to such severe reactions as shock, respiratory failure, and coma.

Other complications include restless sleep, unconsciousness, malnutrition, respiratory illnesses, addiction in a newborn if the mother is addicted, collapse of veins, and increased blood pressure and pulse rate during detoxification.

The heroin user is also subject to violent death because

of his life-style, which may include committing crimes such as breaking and entering, robbery, and burglary. Frequent spans in jail are common, but heroin is available in many penal institutions if the person has the money to purchase it.

METHADONE

medicine, dollies

Various types of treatment for heroin addiction are available. Many cities have methadone clinics. Methadone is a long-acting narcotic that is supposed to be taken orally in an attempt to substitute a "safer" narcotic for heroin. Supposedly it diminishes the craving for heroin as well as blocking the pleasure that heroin produces.

Many persons now attend methadone clinics. Some function well on methadone, but many abuse methadone and heroin together, causing overdose in a number of cases. The methadone withdrawal is also painful, so many people choose to remain on methadone forever.

Other heroin withdrawal methods that feature a total drug-free approach include community drug-abuse programs and residential live-in programs. My feeling is that heroin addiction can be reversed effectively in a large number of persons who are willing to participate in these programs. One of the essential criteria for success is that the user be detoxified and then have asbolutely no contact with her previous peer group. Often moving to another city is necessary, and participation in an ongoing program is essential. The longer an addict can remain sober, the better her chances for complete, lasting success.

Detoxification itself does not stop heroin addiction. A person who is detoxified in a hospital setting and then sent back on the streets will almost invariably return to using heroin or any other drug she has been taking. She must receive intensive therapy and drug-abuse counseling as well as maintain complete drug abstinence to have any chance for success.

DRUGS AND PREGNANCY

Since drugs cause extremely severe problems when they are taken during pregnancy, few studies have been performed directly on pregnant women. Researchers know that many drugs can affect the growth of the fetus and the later mental and physical functioning of the infant. Drugs can also be absorbed by the infant through the mother's milk.

Males and females respond in a similar manner to most drugs, but women metabolize or break down some drugs more slowly than men. In these cases, drugs can be responsible for severe, longer-lasting effects in women.

Serious birth defects, known as congenital birth defects, are those that are usually caused during the first three months of pregnancy (the first trimester). During pregnancy, the fetus receives its nutrition through a blood-vessel linkage to the mother known as the placenta. However, during the first weeks of pregnancy, the placenta is not yet formed and the fetus receives its nutrition from the maternal fluids that surround it.

Almost any drug the mother takes goes first through her bloodstream, affecting her brain, and eventually crossing the placenta into the fetus and the fetal brain. There are very few drugs that do not cross the placenta and reach the fetus. Any drug taken repeatedly that crosses into the placenta will accumulate in the fetus to a level equal to that of the mother's drug level.

It is difficult to say exactly what defects or problems each drug causes in each infant because so many factors are in play. Variables include the amount of drug used, how the drug was taken, how far along the pregnancy is, exposure to other drugs, and if the drug was pure or mixed.

A fetus is particularly sensitive from about the twentieth day after conception through the next two months. After the first three weeks, the embryo's organs start to develop, and drugs at this point can cause severe damage. The amount and severity will depend on what stage of development the organ is at and the amount and type of drug used by the mother.

After this first period, drugs can still retard fetal growth and behavior. For example, it is well known that both cigarette smoking and heroin use often result in below-normal birth weights. Any drug that causes a depression of respiration, as heroin does, can create breathing difficulties in the newborn. If this is prolonged, the baby can suffer brain damage and decreased intellectual functioning.

Some drugs, such as Valium, are known to stay in the newborn's bloodstream for many days and can cause severe problems in the baby's first days. Other drugs, if they are used frequently during pregnancy, can even cause the baby to be born addicted. Frequent barbiturate or heroin use can lead to this situation. The baby may experience a withdrawal syndrome that is similar to an adult's and occasionally even have convulsions.

Alcohol also has severe consequences. "Fetal alcohol syndrome" occurs in the newborns of mothers who are heavy drinkers. It is characterized by abnormal facial features, low I.Q., and growth retardation. At this point it is not known what it is that *exactly* causes this syndrome but it is widely documented.

2

TEENAGE DRUG USE

Every adolescent, as well as every adult, is a unique individual who possesses a distinct personality pattern, previous experiences, psychological conflicts and problems, and individualized thinking mode. Because of the vast differences among individuals, there are many reasons why people first experiment with chemicals and why people continue to use, abuse, and finally become dependent on and/or addicted to drugs and alcohol.

I am going to list some of the more common reasons for using chemicals, then describe these reasons in more detail. Many of these reasons have been given to me by my patients and substantiated by research on drug-using behavior. You will note some overlapping in these causes because much of an adolescent's emotional life is complicated and closely entwined with the environment. These reasons are not necessarily listed in order of importance for any particlar person.

1. peer pressure
2. rebellion against parents and authority
3. feelings of rejection
4. low self-esteem
5. hopelessness

6. excess pressure to perform
7. curiosity and experimentation
8. relief of depression
9. mastery of inhibitions and shyness
10. boredom
11. lack of goals and aimlessness
12. maintaining an image
13. relief of tension and anxiety
14. camouflage of inadequacies
15. "expanded awareness"
16. relief of psychosis
17. relief of pain
18. relief of other stresses

REASONS TEENAGERS USE DRUGS

PEER PRESSURE

Peer pressure, the often-subtle push by one's immediate social group and acquaintances, is one of the chief reasons cited as a cause for using drugs. Many people, not only adolescents, are insecure and exhibit an overwhelming need for the approval of their clique or group. It is human nature to need to know that you are acceptable to a certain degree, but the need for acceptance is perhaps at its greatest during adolescence.

Because of this, many adolescents become followers and will imitate the group in which they wish to be included. One sees this in gangs, high-school sororities and fraternities, and other groups. Many millions of teenagers succumb to peer pressure and initially use drugs to gain the acceptance of the kids who are already on drugs.

As time goes on, the individual becomes more involved in his peer group. If this group has principles that are opposite to the values of other groups, then the adolescent must choose one group over the other. In time a teenager may drop his old friends and associate only with those in

the new peer group. The longer this relationship continues, the less contact there is with the old group and its
values, mores, and goals. He often begins to scorn the
ideas that he used to believe in, perhaps very strongly.
This is the insidious effect that the drugs and the new
friends have on him.

Often the most difficult task parents face is trying to get
their child out of a drug-using peer group. Most parents
who have a child in a drug-abusing peer group will readily
verify this. Peer pressure is such a strong factor that it can
undo the progress made in therapy in a very short period of
time.

The reason outpatient counseling or therapy often fails is
because of this peer influence. If the child only spends a
few hours weekly in treatment but many hours with his
peers, you can imagine how difficult it would be to make
progress toward a sober life, even if the kid is motivated to
do so. Because of this, many psychiatrists feel that the
abuser must be treated in an environment where he is
completely separated from his peer group. I agree that this
is necessary in many situations.

Of equal importance is the fact that the child must become motivated during treatment to drop his peer group if
he is to achieve lasting sobriety. Since adolescent relationships are often extremely intense, it is quite difficult to
convince teens to drop their friends. In many cases, all of a
kid's friends may use drugs, but there is certainly no reason
to drop peers who are drug-free if they are supportive and
stable.

The only solution that seems to work fairly consistently is
if the old peer group can be replaced with a new, positive
group. Asking a teen to drop all his drug-using friends and
not offering him a replacement group is often futile. This
idea is discussed further in the section on community drug-
abuse programs.

Peer pressure is also at least partially responsible for

some of the other reasons listed for drug use, particularly in the areas of social rebellion or protest, experimentation, low self-esteem, and boredom.

REBELLION AGAINST PARENTS AND AUTHORITY

An adolescent rebelling against parents and other authority figures is certainly not a new phenomenon. Many of you reading this book probably remember going through that period yourselves. It is part of the common adolescent experience. A teenager normally tries to develop a sense of autonomy and independence. In many ways, it is much more difficult today than it was in the past.

In the past young people would rebel only to a certain extent against their parents. Using drugs was not usually an option open to them, although alcohol was freely available. But most teens would rebel by having different opinions on subjects, arguing with their parents, staying out late, and having a different dress code. All of this is still with us, but drug abuse is now added to the list.

Over the last twenty years the severity of this sort of rebellion has increased. Physical fighting, physical injury, running away, stealing parents' possessions, and verbal abuse have become common. And many parents have become more abusive to their offspring. Frequently this is because of intense provocation; other times it is indicative of the parents' own psychological difficulties.

And it is not only parents who have rebellion directed toward them. Ask public school teachers about the abuses that have been heaped upon them by many students. Coaches, police officers, employers have all been stunned by the rebellion that they have witnessed from adolescents.

Rebellion is the way people can show their displeasure with someone. Adolescents become very irritable while hormonal and psychological changes take place in their bodies and minds. They become easily upset, angry, hostile, and resentful. They often see their parents and the teachers as the enemy.

A classic way to rebel against someone is to practice values and life-style that are the opposite of the person being rebelled against. Since most parents are certainly against their children using drugs, a perfect rebellion is to go out and get high. Some adolescents do not even try to hide the fact from their parents. They want them to know that they are rebelling.

Rebellion, once a relatively short-lived situation, can easily become the first step toward drug abuse and drug addiction. It can eventually estrange the adolescent from her family to the point of her leaving home permanently or damaging the relationship beyond repair. For these reasons therapy is often indicated at the beginning of the rebellious period. The less time that the family has lived under a severely rebellious period, the better the prognosis for resolution of the family problems.

FEELINGS OF REJECTION

Many teenagers have an intense expectation of being rejected. This feeling comes from a combination of their own past experiences and the hormonal and psychological changes that they are undergoing. Practically no one escapes the experience of being rejected by a certain person or group of people as he is growing up.

As the young adolescent goes through a number of changes both emotionally and physically, he begins to question whether he is acceptable, attractive, and in general okay. Since many, if not most, people at this stage have little skill in giving personal compliments or in sharing their feelings with others, they have no one to answer these questions for them.

The easiest way to avoid these feelings of nonacceptance is to dismiss their relevance entirely. Instead of worrying if one is too short, too tall, physically unattractive, a bore, or just generally not right, it is much easier not to think about it at all. Once a teen finds out that drugs will block these feelings completely while he is high, he will turn to drugs as the most expedient way of dealing with uncomfortable personal issues.

Rejection, or fear of rejection, can come from many experiences. If the adolescent has received a lot of rejection from those close to him—his family, friends, and classmates—he will be even more keenly sensitive about himself. Unfortunately, many parents seem not to speak to their children except to correct or scold them.

These children will grow up to anticipate rejection from almost everyone. They don't expect anyone ever to find them worthwhile, and their self-esteem is low. Communication with a child—any child—should focus on attributes more than deficiencies. This is the way a person builds self-confidence. And the more self-confidence a teenager has, the less likely he is to use drugs and the more likely he is to continue to see himself in a good light and attempt to continue to be productive.

LOW SELF-ESTEEM

This is one characteristic that is seen in almost all persons who abuse drugs. Many adolescents who are interviewed will admit that they have feelings of low self-esteem and worthlessness, and little self-confidence. Others often deny these feelings and attempt to overcompensate for them. Even their psychological test results show lowered self-esteem.

Obviously low self-esteem is often related to feelings of rejection as well hopelessness, depression, boredom, and shyness. It is the most common component of adolescent depression. Young people who do not overcome these feelings are open to a much higher risk of drug and alcohol abuse, self-destructive behavior, school and work failure, marital and family problems, and severe depression and suicide.

One way for these kids to avoid feeling bad about themselves is to get high and ignore all unpleasant thoughts or emotional states. But once the high wears off, the feelings return, and the quickest way to obtain relief is to get high again. Thus the vicious cycle begins.

Low self-esteem is such an important issue that many self-help books have been written presenting the issue as the central problem in many life situations. There is no doubt that a real improvement in feelings about oneself is absolutely necessary for any long-lasting therapeutic change.

Improvement in self-esteem is one of the main benefits of supportive drug-abuse programs. The support and acceptance of others in the program make participants feel better about themselves, and they tend to depend on the program during this period because it makes them feel happier. Programs that are exclusively confrontive, without being supportive, have a much lower success rate, which is quite understandable.

The same holds true for families. Those that show support and love fare better than those that only communicate their dissatisfactions. It is much easier to change in a loving, caring environment than in a hostile one.

HOPELESSNESS

Hopelessness is one of the most frustrating experiences a human can endure. It is related to severely low self-esteem and lack of positive experiences and is often sensed as general despair. People who repeatedly find themselves in untenable situations develop a feeling of hopelessness. If nothing positive happens, they begin to feel that nothing will change, and then hopelessness sets in.

Obviously drug abuse has a perfect opportunity to develop in this situation. Relief from this uncomfortable state is desired, and drugs seem to be the perfect answer. But once dependency on drugs has developed, then the hopelessness will return in an even greater degree.

Many drug and alcohol programs have a spiritual aspect to them that is very helpful in dealing with feelings of hopelessness. They help participants develop faith in themselves, and this can be of enormous help in combating the hopelessness. When a teenager hears people in the program tell how hopeless they once felt and how they were able to overcome it with the help of the group (and possibly therapy), the adolescent realizes that his feelings are not so unique, or incurable.

Many people need immediate hospitalization when they reach this state of despair: the risk of suicide is high when feelings of hopelessness are so strong. If someone in your family is expressing these feelings, seek professional help immediately. You should understand that kids can become severely depressed even when it seems as though there's no apparent reason to feel this way. Often people's feelings do not translate outwardly, and their lives may appear directly opposite to their emotional states.

Families with an optimistic view of life, that are not overly concerned with failure and financial burdens and that share a spiritual life seem less likely to have a family member develop these hopeless feelings. Furthermore, families are at lower risk if they have the ability to communicate their feelings and concerns with each other openly.

EXCESS PRESSURE TO PERFORM

Many families could be described as overachievers. In these families there is an excessive emphasis placed on performance in areas such as academic achievement, athletics, beauty, or just "doing everything right." At least one person in these families has "achieved" much in life, at least by parental standards. The situation is worse when both parents feel this way.

I am not referring to the feeling that most parents have of wanting to see their children grow up to be productive members of society. I am speaking of a strong push to have the child come out number one in almost everything he attempts to do. This is an enormous task that the child may feel obligated to perform to please his parents. But it may be impossible because of a number of circumstances. For example, a boy may not be as coordinated as his father or as popular as his brother. A girl may not be as pretty as her mother or sister or as gifted academically. Adding the stress of normal adolescent development to this excessive pressure, you have a situation that can produce overwhelming anxiety. Again, drugs are a way to relieve uncomfortable feelings. In addition, rebellion is apt to be likely if the pressure is unbearable. I have seen straight-A students rebel and turn to drugs for relief. Their grades have fallen to Ds and Fs in as short a time as one semester.

Perhaps the best tactic is to motivate the youngster to perform at his best level *for himself* rather than to please anyone else. It is the same concept used in getting a kid off drugs—one can only really stay off drugs for oneself.

CURIOSITY AND EXPERIMENTATION

Many adolescents are curious about a number of things, drugs being just one of them. It is apparent that the vast majority of teenagers try at least some chemical during their teenage years. Many do this not for rebellion, avoidance, or any of the reasons mentioned previously but simply out of curiosity. Hopefully for these teens the experimentation will end once their curiosity is satisfied. For many it does not.

I have heard literally hundreds of teens tell me and my

staff that they just wanted to see how it feels. They enjoyed the euphoria and continued to get high. Eventually they began to experiment with other drugs because they were curious about the different highs they would experience.

Curiosity itself is not the problem; it is the avenue into which it is directed. One way to deal with this issue is with early education. I caution parents not to leave this education to the schools but to undertake it themselves so they know that it has really been accomplished. Developing your child's interests in other things may help her satisfy her curiosity in a much healthier and safer way.

RELIEF OF DEPRESSION

Depression is related both to low self-esteem and to feelings of hopelessness. It is a state that most of us have experienced at one time or another. Sometimes it has been in response to a tragic situation, and perhaps this should best be described as grief rather than depression.

Depression is a state of sadness that can have many causes. In the adolescent years it is often caused by family tension, rejection by family or peers, feelings of inadequacy, pressure to excel, stress, lack of goals, and for no apparent reason at all. In the latter situation, the reason usually becomes clear once therapy is begun.

Depression is a very treatable illness, but many people, not only adolescents, tend to medicate themselves instead with legal or illegal stimulants; amphetamines (speed) are the drug of choice. The stimulant gives them a false sense of well-being and energy. Consequently they feel less depressed temporarily.

Other kids report that they do not feel any better when they are high, just different. This is another kind of relief of depression by an alteration of state of mind. Some teens report that drugs make them feel worse when they are depressed, yet they take them anyway.

Part of the problem is that many adolescents have the clinical illness of depression yet do not sense the depression like most of us do. Some typical symptoms of depressed states, besides the feeling of depression, are sleep disturbances (increased or decreased amount of sleep), changes in appetite, loss of interest, increased irritability, frequent arguments, loss of sexual interest, decreased performance at work or school, and fatigue.

MASTERY OF INHIBITIONS AND SHYNESS

Adolescents often tend to question their own acceptability, as mentioned previously. They wonder if their social skills will cause them to be rejected or accepted. Many adolescents fret about this to the point that they become inhibited, shy, and socially self-conscious. Their fears center around saying the wrong thing, appearing foolish or dumb, being excluded from a group, and being rejected by peers of their own sex or the opposite sex.

Since drugs tend to loosen inhibitions, they are partially successful in helping an adolescent deal with these fears. Many kids tell me they can say things and be more relaxed when they are high, because if they are rejected then they can always blame it on the fact that they were high and not in control of themselves. Many teens begin to depend on the drug to give them courage. It can easily lead to the point that they will not deal with any frustrating situation unless they are stoned. And this is exactly how psychological dependency on chemicals develops.

Inhibitions and shyness are related to low self-esteem. As the person develops better feelings about himself and finds himself acceptable to himself, then the shyness diminishes. He no longer needs to be accepted by peers to feel good because he truly knows that he is okay. Similarly, the effects of peer pressure are less.

Practically everyone has been rejected by someone at

some time. Many people bounce right back and go on to the next person or group. But some teens react by withdrawing to a large degree from newcomers and strangers. They may be open with their familiar peer group but very shy and inhibited when faced with new people. They are simply using a defense mechanism against the possibility of going through the hurt of being rejected again.

BOREDOM

Another often mentioned reason for getting high is boredom. Teenagers complain about boredom very frequently. It is interesting to note that teens I have treated from cities that are large enough to offer many activities, such as Houston, Los Angeles, and New York, complain about boredom as frequently as teenagers from cities with very small populations and few diversions.

Part of the problem is that outside interests have not been promoted by the family or that the adolescent is depressed and has lost interest in things. Furthermore, once a teen uses drugs frequently, she becomes almost exclusively interested in getting high and the associated lifestyle.

The same phenomenon is seen in adult substance abusers. Their whole lives may revolve around drugs. Once drugs are removed from their lives, they really have no idea what to do with all their free time. We have found it necessary to set up special groups in our hospital programs to deal with leisure-time activities.

Most teens lead lives that are similar once they get into daily usage of drugs. This involves getting high, listening to music, perhaps having sex. Little else is really done. Since they cannot concentrate well, school appears very boring, as do most jobs. Doing the same thing every day, whether it is getting high, working at a job, or taking care of a home, can become monotonous. But the only thing a drug-using teen cares about is drugs, so there is no variety to the schedule, no special interests or pastimes that are enjoyable. Without this, life is fairly dull for anyone.

Boredom is something parents need to be aware of. If your child seems bored, you need to take time to expose him to the many different activities that he or she could enjoy. In the process you may find new interests for yourself. It seems to me that the more interests anyone has, the more fulfilling and satisfying his whole life will be.

LACK OF GOALS AND AIMLESSNESS

This area is closely related to boredom. Many adolescents have no particular goals in life. They tend to let life direct them where it may. This can lead to depression, boredom, and even hopelessness.

Although I do not feel that an adolescent should necessarily have his whole life planned out, I do feel that some immediate plans for the near future are important. If a person can decide on a particular goal, develop a plan for achieving the goal, then expend energy and willpower in working toward this goal, he will feel better about his capabilities when the goal is reached. If the initial plan fails but he has alternative plans that work, he also learns that perseverance is a worthy virtue. Even failure can have its reward. Kids can learn that the importance of making the attempt as well as of the actual achievement.

But many, many adolescents are completely blocked when asked what they want out of life. They say they just want to be able to get high. This certainly seems like a small goal, given the opportunities that are available to teenagers throughout the country. Others on drugs seem to want a lot of material comforts, particularly without having to work for them.

Marijuana is particularly well known for producing an "amotivational syndrome." This is a state that is characterized by lack of goals, lack of motivation, and general lack of interest in anything besides getting high. Other drugs can cause a similar state of mind. Setting goals and then working toward them is one of the last things that someone who is in this state of mind will think of.

MAINTAINING AN IMAGE

Maintaining an image or external facade is important to many teenagers. For boys the "macho," tough-guy image is common. Girls may present this image or one of seduction to society. Other fronts may also be used. Whatever the image is, it serves a function of defense for the teenager.

The child is usually defending against letting certain people get close to him, or she is identifying with a certain group. Adolescents may try to keep people far enough from their inner self so as to not be a threat to their internal security. Often the people who are kept away are the parents or other authority figures.

The image can develop as a result of peer pressure, rebellion against parental or societal standards, or attempts at independence and autonomy. Some facades are unconsciously used to keep attention focused on the person because the only way he knows to gain attention is by negative behavior.

This is often one of the difficult parts of therapy. The therapy team must penetrate this defensive wall and help the child let down the barriers before any real changes can take place. To do this means that trust must be developed between the user and his therapist. Therapists who obviously side with the parents will have an impossible situation on their hands. They must try to take no sides in the therapy and to be very supportive and understanding of the teenager in their individual sessions.

Often a very tough external image is a defense against more tender feelings. If a kid feels unloved, she may present an image of someone who seems unlovable. Many people seem to be able to sense anger easily, but feelings such as love, closeness, and caring are harder to experience. Drugs are often used to relieve some of the tension that is generated from feeling anger so frequently and strongly.

RELIEF OF TENSION AND ANXIETY

Many experiences of both teenagers and adults generate tension and anxiety. Many people who are in a depressed state also feel anxious. Adolsecent fears of rejection, parental strife, heterosexual dating, and low self-esteem all can lead to an anxiety state.

Tension can be measured clinically by the use of biofeedback machines. Practically all the adolescents we treat for drugs show tension levels above the normal range. Almost all of them can learn how to control anxiety and tension consciously without having to use an artificial chemical.

Being anxious is a very uncomfortable state. We have all experienced it at one time or another. It took us a number of years to learn how to deal with it effectively. The process of dealing with it many times teaches us how to relax and function during times of greater than usual stress.

But people who take drugs generally do not learn how to deal with anxiety because the drugs will blot out the uncomfortable feelings temporarily. Consequently they develop no skills in functioning and coping with anxiety. Their thresholds for anxiety are lowered. This clearly plays a part in the vicious cycle of drugs. If you feel anxious, get high. When the drug wears off and the anxiety returns, get high again. This is the mode of operation of most frequent drug abusers.

Many kids in treatment initially feel worse when they enter into the treatment process because their crutch—the drugs—has been removed. They must now deal with the tensions, anxieties, and frustrations that they have been avoiding through the use of drugs. But there is no other way. They have to throw away the crutch sooner or later if they are ever going to be able to deal with life. The kids who are not willing to try to walk without this crutch are the ones who drop out of treatment and return to using drugs or alcohol.

CAMOUFLAGE OF INADEQUACIES

Some adolescents use drugs to camouflage such problems as poor school performance, learning disabilities, reading problems, and social inadequacies. Groups of kids using drugs all seem somewhat similar to each other because they share the same activity. There is no test to perform well, no particular skill associated with getting high. Anyone can do it, so inadequacies are not so apparent in the group setting.

Academic or social deficiencies usually lead to a teenager feeling bad about himself, lack of confidence, anxiety, and even hopelessness. But these shortcomings can be overcome if the child's self-esteem is improved. One technique is to help the adolescent focus on his attributes as a human being rather than on his deficiencies. In reality, there is always someone who can do something better than we can do it. But many kids have qualities that they are not even aware of. Perhaps the emphasis in their family has been on athletic or academic achievement. Their skills may lie more in the areas of music, sharing and communicating with others, or other more creative activities.

One way the drug-abuse groups are effective is in letting people in the group know that they are appreciated for who they are rather than for any particular achievements in a certain area. Someone who can show that she cares may be much more important to other people than someone who can perform well in school or sports. Once kids can rearrange their priorities along these lines, they often begin to realize that they are no less important than anyone else.

"EXPANDED AWARENESS"

This is a term left over from the 1960s. At that time much emphasis was placed on drugs such as the hallucinogens that would "expand one's awareness." This meant to have a hallucinatory experience with an increase in visual and auditory sensations as well as to let your mind think in a psychotic fashion. Some people felt they had enormous intellectual insights during these periods, but this belief is questioned by many researchers in the field.

Once again some of the hallucinogens, particularly "acid" (LSD), are back with us. There has been a large increase in the use of acid by the teenage population since about 1977. Unfortunately, the consequences can be a life-long tragedy. I have covered this in some detail in the section on hallucinogens.

The more tragic side effects are permanent psychosis and "flashbacks." These drugs are notorious for causing severe feelings of paranoia. Rather than resulting in an enlightened individual, the usual picture is one of a confused, paranoid, somewhat emotionally fragile and unstable adolescent who has difficulty with his thought processes. Because of this he has problems relating both to peers and to adults. He often feels isolated and estranged from his social circle.

A safer way to expand one's awareness is to learn how to listen, think, feel, and experience situations with an open mind. This may not be as exciting or as easy as taking a hallucinogen, but the ultimate results can be much more satisfying.

RELIEF OF PSYCHOSIS

Some adolescents, albeit a great minority, develop a psychotic illness. This is often not known by the family, and only an experienced clinician may be able to detect the condition. Psychotic experiences can include visual and auditory hallucinations, delusions, and illusions, but they very often exist without these symptoms. They are marked by turmoil, a particular mode of thinking, a high degree of ambivalence, and change and lability in the person's emotions.

Because the symptoms cause so much tension and overwhelming anxiety to the child who is in this state, he is often seeking relief from this very uncomfortable mood. He finds that some drugs, particularly sedatives, marijuana, and pain relievers, cause a lessening of tension by their sedative effects. These drugs are not what we call antipsychotic drugs. They do not reverse the bizarre thought processes, but they do diminish the associated anxiety to some degree. People in this situation are usually in need of correct treatment for their psychological state of mind. There are medications—the major tranquilizers or "antipsychotic drugs"—that are very helpful in treating such psychosis, especially if they are combined with appropriate therapy.

Other drugs can make a psychosis much worse. Amphetamines, cocaine, and the hallucinogenic drugs often tend to worsen an already psychotic state. Since hallucinogens are psychomimetic drugs—they produce a temporary psychotic state—you can see how destructive they would be to someone who is already having problems with thinking clearly.

If a psychosis is suspected because a teenager is exhibiting bizarre thinking patterns and strange behavior, it is best to seek professional help with an experienced adolescent psychiatrist as soon as possible. The usual time for onset of this illness is late adolescence, but it can occur earlier.

RELIEF OF PAIN

Some people become dependent on drugs because they were first taking them by prescription for relief of physical pain. The pain relievers are usually termed "analgesics." The stronger the medication for relieving pain, the more addicting is its potential. The majority of people who begin abusing drugs in this fashion are usually older. They have either injured themselves or developed an illness that produces some pain, such as back problems, arthritis, or other joint or muscle pains.

The other type of pain that people are trying to relieve is emotional. Many of the situations described previously could be termed emotional pain. Loneliness, rejection, depression, and other sad, empty states place a teenager in an emotionally painful state, and drugs or alcohol are often used in an attempt to relieve this uncomfortable condition.

There are various methods that can help a person who has physical pain, such as biofeedback and neurotone. For both physical and emotional pain, treatment is usually indicated, either on an outpatient or an inpatient basis.

RELIEF OF OTHER STRESSES

Although this has been covered in the previous sections, it is best to mention again some of the adolescent stresses that a teenage drug user is trying to avoid. These include family tension and discord, fear of rejection by family and peers, feeling of real or imagined inadequacies, learning disabilities, fear of heterosexual rejection, fear of latent homosexuality, depression, hopelessness, aimlessness, and the ever-present peer pressure.

Again, the relief brought by drugs is a temporary cure, because the pressures and associated feelings will return when the drugs wear off. The only real cure is to cease drug use completely and work through the psychological problems. Once the problems are really dealt with, the need for using drugs diminishes accordingly. That means entering a treatment program, laying down the crutch of drugs, and going through the pain and discomfort of looking clearly at oneself and growing through a process of intensive therapy.

HIGH RISK FACTORS LEADING TO DRUG USE

If any of the situations listed below are prevalent in an adolescent's environment, then there is a strong likelihood of drug use. A combination of several or all of these factors is a danger signal.

> peer pressure groups
> chaotic or separated family
> dissatisfying or unhappy family relationships
> cigarette use by teenager
> parental use of 1 pack or more of cigarettes daily
> parental use of tranquilizers (prescribed or otherwise)
> regular alcohol use by parents
> sibling usage of drugs
> no active religious life
> low self-esteem
> lack of goals and aimlessness
> lack of participation in social events

DEFENSE MECHANISMS

Kids who abuse drugs, although they may not have actual psychiatric illness, tend to use a number of defense mechanisms frequently. These defenses help to allay anxiety, and even the use of drugs can be looked upon as another defense mechanism in that it also may help relieve anxiety.

Defense mechanisms are very specific processes that people use to relieve themselves from emotional conflict and to produce freedom from anxiety. A defense mechanism is an unconscious working of the mind, although one can consciously employ it. All humans use defense mechanisms at one time or another, but the frequent, almost continual use of specific defenses is seen in neurotic conditions.

There are many defense mechanisms that teenagers can employ. These include the following: avoidance, compensation, conversion, denial, displacement, dissociation, idealization, identification, incorporation, introjection, projection, rationalization, reaction formation, repression, sublimation, substitution, symbolization, and undoing.

When the defense mechanisms are no longer able to keep anxiety under control, a neurotic or psychotic illness may develop. An example of a neurotic illness would be anxiety neurosis, in which an unbearable state of anxiety exists. Another neurotic illness would be obsessive-compulsive neurosis, in which the person is plagued by repetitive impulses to perform certain acts, such as hand washing, counting, or checking situations out repeatedly.

When defense mechanisms of a certain nature are prominent, such as projection, a psychotic illness may develop. In this situation there is a loss of contact with reality; distortion of perceptions, including hallucinations and delusions; regressed behavior; and bizarre thinking.

The defense mechanisms that seem to be used commonly by drug abusers are avoidance, compulsions, denial, displacement, identification, projection, rationalization, reaction formation, repression, and sublimation. Other mechanisms may also be used, but these are the most frequently seen.

AVOIDANCE

One common defense that drug users employ is the unconscious avoidance of any unpleasant situation. They often try

to structure their environment to avoid anyone pointing
out their aberrant behavior, deficiencies, or life-style. They
may avoid school by skipping and also avoid social interac-
tions in which they might feel inadequate or rejected; they
tend, therefore, to stay within the drug-using group that
accepts their behavior. They also avoid situations in which
they may fail, thus indicating that they might be less capable and potent than they wish others to believe.

COMPULSIONS

Many kids who use drugs exhibit compulsive mechanisms
and behavior, and this is particularly true in those who are
addicted. They sense an inner drive to repeat certain behaviors such as getting high, even in the absence of any
physical addiction. Their compulsive urges may not be limited to the act of taking the drugs but may include urges to
lie, steal, cheat, or exhibit other antisocial behavior.

DENIAL

This is another unconscious defense mechanism that assists
the person to avoid anxiety or conflict by denying a
thought, feeling, wish, need, or any reality that is consciously intolerable. This is a very frequent finding among
the drug users I have treated. They have a high resistance
to allowing themselves to accept any uncomfortable feelings, particularly if the acceptance of these feelings would
diminish their own sense of importance.

Many adolescents start treatment in a state of total denial, to the extent that they will deny that they even use
drugs or that drugs cause them any difficulties in their
relationships with parents or peers. Other denied issues
are that drugs are affecting their lives, that they cannot
control their urge to get high, or that they ought to consider changing the direction in which their lives are
headed.

Denial of feelings such as anger, hate, rejection, love, sadness, and caring is common. Feelings that produce a new or uncomfortable emotional state are the ones that are most commonly denied. Many users, especially those who have been involved with drugs for some time, have become so out of touch with their feelings that they are actually incapable of experiencing normal feelings.

DISPLACEMENT

This defense is one of unconsciously transferring or "displacing" an emotion from its original object to a more acceptable substitute. For the drug user, the substitute that might be more acceptable is the drug.

As an example of how this works, a child may have a high degree of dependence on another person, perhaps a parent or sibling. But these unconscious feelings of dependency may be unacceptable to him. They may make him feel weak, unacceptable, even make him feel fear that he is homosexual. He may then displace his dependency needs onto drugs, which are psychologically more acceptable for him at this point.

Another displacement might be to replace the need to belong to an identifiable group such as his family by a need to belong to a gang or peer group. The child's need to belong to the family may be unconsciously uncomfortable because it indicates that he is not as autonomous or independent as he would like everyone to believe; thus the displacement to the peer group.

IDENTIFICATION

This occurs when the adolescent unconsciously identifies herself with another person or even a group. This identification with another person makes the child more like the other person, thus improving the chances of acceptance and diminishing the chances of being rejected.

This is the defense mechanism that is much in force in the area of peer pressure. Identification with a particular person or with the mores of a whole group is a very powerful defense mechanism (please review the section on peer pressure). It is one of the reasons that treatment can be such a difficult process. Part of the task of the therapist is to diminish this intensive identification with the wrong kind of model and to replace the identification with a positive role model.

PROJECTION

This is the unconscious mechanism by which a teen rejects an unacceptable emotion within himself and attributes, or projects, it to others. He then believes that the other person has these unacceptable feelings or emotions.

This is a common defense mechanism in certain psychotic illnesses such as schizophrenia. It can also be found in nonpsychotic persons as well. One example of how it might exhibit itself in the drug user is that an adolescent user who has a high degree of anger and hatred toward one parent may project that the parent hates him and then use drugs to block the uncomfortable feeling he has that his parent hates him. Some users project all their unacceptable feelings and thoughts onto "society." It is "society" that has it in for them—the values, rules, and laws of society seem to be established to make the user's life unhappy.

RATIONALIZATION

With this commonly used defense, the adolescent attempts to justify her thoughts, feelings, and actions in order to make them consciously acceptable, or tolerable, to herself. Many people use this technique; it is not limited to drug users by any means. But users of drugs employ this defense quite frequently.

Some common rationalizations I hear are "My drug usage doesn't hurt anyone," "I can handle drugs because

I'm stronger than other people," "The only thing wrong with my using drugs is that they are illegal," "No one cares about me anyway," "I don't have a problem—I can stop anytime," and "The things they say about drugs are just to scare you." Countless other rationalizations are also used to justify drug abuse.

Many adolescent rationalizations seem almost plausible to some parents. But the parents need to look at the loopholes inherent in these rationalizations. The more articulate the adolescent, the more difficult it is to refute these false reasonings. But the rationalization is usually based on an idea or assumption the basis of which is false.

REACTION FORMATION

This is a situation in which attitudes and behaviors are employed that are the opposite of impulses the person has in his conscious or unconscious mind. The outward behavior is presented to counteract the opposite, unwanted thoughts.

If the teenager has been raised to lead a moral, religious life, the opposite type of life-style may develop. This may be a reaction formation that is used as a rebellion against parental standards and ideals. His peers may be opposed to these parental values, so the alignment may be both identification with peers and reaction formation against the now-unacceptable parental standards.

On the other hand, many kids will act overly solicitous and caring about someone, for instance an invalid parent, to overcompensate for the resentment and anger they feel at having their time consumed entirely by caring for this person. This is a common type of reaction formation and is usually completely unconscious.

REPRESSION

Repression is another unconscious mechanism by which a person removes unacceptable ideas, feelings, or impulses from consciousness. It can also be used to prevent these ideas, feelings, and impulses from ever reaching consciousness in the first place. A similar mechanism is suppression, but suppression is a conscious mechanism, whereas repression works completely outside the awareness of the person.

Repression is a universal defense mechanism that is used by everyone, to some extent, every day. The drug abuser uses it both in her normal functioning and as a part of her mode of making her drug-using behavior acceptable to herself. She represses any ideas or feelings that her actions might be unacceptable, thus allowing her to behave in a manner that is not normally acceptable to her; in this manner taking drugs, stealing, or other dissocial behavior becomes unacceptable.

When repression fails to work adequately, the teen may experience a severe loss of self-esteem as the unacceptable thoughts and feelings she has previously pushed out of awareness now return to plague her conscious thoughts. Depression usually follows, and this is an optimal time to motivate the child to begin treatment, as she would like to find relief from the highly uncomfortable state of depression.

SUBLIMATION

This is a process by which a person unconsciously diverts unacceptable impulses into more socially acceptable channels. An example of normal sublimation would be a person who has a high degree of unacceptable aggression choosing boxing as a professional career, boxing being more acceptable than getting into physical fights with friends and acquaintances.

At first glance it appears that sublimation is not in force in drug users, as they are behaving in a socially unacceptable manner. But the behavior of using drugs may be unacceptable to parents and authority but not to the peer group. A user may have an unacceptable urge to fight, be a loner, withdraw from friends, or lose control of himself. He may sublimate these urges into taking drugs because it is more acceptable in his group and the drugs act to relieve his urges artificially if he chooses ones with the correct pharmaceutical effects.

3

PARENT PREVENTIVE TECHNIQUES

Jimmy is in jail. As I write this chapter I wonder how many other people will have to go through the same pain and suffering that Jimmy and his family have endured.

Jimmy turned eighteen barely three months ago. His mother called me this morning. She was crying, very upset, and felt hopeless. She kept saying to me, "Maybe I could have prevented it. Maybe I raised him wrong."

Jimmy's story is, unfortunately, not uncommon. He started drinking a small amount of beer on weekends when he was thirteen. By the time he was fourteen, he was smoking marijuana two or three times a week. He was still able to function in school, but his attitude and behavior were showing the early signs of changing.

At fifteen he was expelled from school for possession of pot and pills. After returning and again being caught for possession, he quit school upon finishing ninth grade. He refused to get a job, and his parents tried to get him to attend the local drug-abuse program, but they were unsuccessful. "I don't have a drug problem. All my friends use more drugs than I do," he told them. His parents finally gave up trying to get him to change.

But now he is in the county jail. He was arrested three days ago for breaking into an apartment and stealing a TV, silverware, and some money. He told his parents that he did not have enough money to buy the drugs he needed. He had been breaking into homes and apartments for over a year.

And, believe it or not, his mother says he still denies that drugs are the problem. It seems so obvious to anyone reading this, but not to Jimmy. This is one of the alterations in thinking that drugs cause—inability to acknowledge the difference between right and wrong. He has reluctantly agreed to come to the hospital for treatment at this point.

Is there anything parents can do to decrease the possibility of their children using drugs? Many parents see the expanding epidemic of drug abuse as a hopeless situation. They have observed a phenomenon develop over the last fifteen to twenty years that initially seemed to be contained in a particular group— the "hippies" and "flower children" of the 1960s, or the jazz musicians of the 40s and 50s. As the media reported about drugs in a less dramatic fashion in the 1970s, many people mistakenly thought the drug problem was diminishing and even disappearing.

Nothing could be further from the truth. The prevalence of drug use has spread from the colleges of the 60s into the high schools, junior or middle schools, grade schools, and work situations. The use of drugs has finally reached a pandemic degree which affects even the smallest villages in the country in contrast to being an exclusively urban problem originally.

In recent years, particularly the last four, parent groups have been organized across the country, started by parents who are particularly interested in prevention to decrease future drug use in their community and in stopping problems before they start. Their focus is on the younger child and high-risk preadolescent and teenager. The parent groups, often called parent awareness groups or parent peer groups, are loosely associated with each other and may vary in their area of interest, depending on the problems that are unique to their community. The groups gather from weekly to monthly, often in schools and churches, and share ideas and research, present guest speakers, and plan actions to take in their homes and communities.

I have spoken to many leaders of this movement and feel that their efforts will be effective to a large degree, especially for the children of the parents in the group. Many of us specializing in the treatment of drug abuse feel that the problem is here to stay, at least for many years. Because of subtle (and often overt) condoning of drugs by television programming and sports and entertainment figures, attitudes have been much more accepting of "casual" drug use. "Casual use" in young adolescents is a dangerous situation, as it is difficult for an unformed psyche to cope with the effects of drugs, and kids will often progress to heavier use of chemicals. A concerted effort by literally millions of people over many years will be required to alter the conception that young people can handle drugs.

Because of the probability of drugs remaining in our culture, prevention becomes all the more important. When I speak of prevention I am referring to individual families and relatively small groups, although as the concept spreads to more communities, we may see prevention on a larger, national scale. For example, in Atlanta, Georgia, there are approximately sixty parent groups in the metropolitan area. A list of central offices of parent groups and other organizations can be found at the end of this book.

What techniques do the parents use? How can they make their children understand that drugs are dangerous? How do they obtain drug information, disseminate it, and teach their community leaders about it? I will attempt to answer these and other questions in this chapter, as well as deal with some of the reasons teenagers use drugs and offer some ideas to help parents understand and deal with these problems.

ORGANIZING A PARENT PEER GROUP

Perhaps the most difficult task in the parent-group movement is getting started. Usually the process begins when two or more parents realize they have a serious drug problem in their own home or among their children's friends and acquaintances. After writing to the groups that are listed at the end of the book, they have contacted as many neighbors as possible and held informal meetings to discuss the problem. Many parents initially deny the overall problem or refuse to believe their child may be involved. There is generally a moderate to high drop-out rate initially, usually of the parents who are uninterested and deny or avoid the facts.

It takes some time before a parents' group really evolves, and many organizations have the frustrating experience of seeing new faces at meetings but not the people who were present at the last gathering. This is partly because the program may not be stimulating; the speeches may be irrelevant, and there may be a lack of interest or a feeling of hopelessness on the part of many parents. These problems are solved with time, experience, reevaluation of the approaches that are being used to reach people, presentation by experts in the field, perseverance, and publicity.

There are many techniques available to form a functioning, effective parent group, and I will attempt to present ideas that various parents have used successfully.

LITERATURE

The first step is self-education. One must become familiar with many aspects of the drug culture both to understand the problem and to conceptualize a plan of action. A list of reading material is provided at the end of this book. Certain treatment centers specializing in drug and alcohol abuse also have literature available. However, it is best to read this material carefully, as some "drug-abuse programs" are pro drug use and publish very deceptive pamphlets that are often designed to encourage parents to allow their children to experiment with marijuana and other drugs. Federal and state governments also provide pamphlets, but as the information in them is often incomplete or out of date, they must also be checked thoroughly.

Be wary of outdated material. For example, much of the research conducted on marijuana just eight to ten years ago is quite inaccurate, due to faulty research methods as well as low-grade (low THC content, the most potent psychoactive substance in marijuana) marijuana being used. The marijuana on the streets during the last few years is of a much higher potency—has a much higher THC content— with correspondingly more serious side effects.

As you become involved in a program of self-education about the drug problem, you might start cultivating a few other concerned parents who are interested in drug abuse and share the material with them. This is a common method to organize the "core" of the parent peer group.

PARAPHERNALIA

As you read the various pamphlets, avenues will be pointed out that you will want to pursue. Visual aids are particularly important in impressing a group, and one technique parents use is to collect all the newspaper and magazine articles about drugs that they can find, especially as they relate to their own community. As you are doing this, go to the local "head shops" (department stores, specialty shops, and record shops that sell drug paraphernalia). They are abundant, and you will be surprised at the ingenuity of the manufacturers of the paraphernalia. Buy as much of it as you can. Stash cans, designed to hide drugs, are made to resemble legal merchandise, such as Coca-Cola cans and beer cans, and have a top that screws off with a "stash" space inside. Unsuspecting parents would simply assume a soft-drink container was left in their child's room. Other containers are available to hide small amounts of drugs and other paraphernalia.

An excellent brochure is available from CICOM (Citizens for Informed Choices on Marijuana), 300 Broad St., Stanford, Ct. 06901.

Also sold legally in these stores as well as in grocery and convenience stores are rolling papers to roll "joints" of marijuana. Other paraphernalia includes "roach clips" (to hold marijuana joints), "coke spoons" (to hold cocaine for sniffing), cocaine vials for storage, and pipes to smoke marijuana, hashish, and even heroin. Pipes can be electric, air-driven, chamber, or water pipes.

Many other items are available, often in disguised form. Pens that are actually marijuana roach clips, "bongs" and "carburetors" used to force large amounts of smoke into the user's lungs, and even masks to capture all the smoke in the nasal passages and throat are legally for sale.

Also available is the paraphernalia for harder drugs, such as cocaine and heroin. Some examples are kits (legal) for planting, growing, and harvesting various drugs; for producing, manufacturing, processing, and preparing illegal drugs. In addition, one can buy equipment to test drugs and adulterate and dilute chemicals (such as to "cut" cocaine or heroin for a higher resale profit). Paraphernalia is obviously big business.

Do not forget to buy copies of the prodrug magazines such as *High Times*. You will be amazed at how plentiful copies are. There are even prodrug comic books being sold to five-year-olds. Get some!

I am mentioning paraphernalia at this point as it is an important area of information for the parent peer group and will be dealt with further later in this chapter.

SIGNS OF DRUG USE

By this point you have amassed quite a bit of information on how prevalent drug abuse is throughout the country. You must have some knowledge of how to detect drug usage, both for your own information and to share with others. I have listed in Chapter 1 the most common signs and symptoms of drug abuse. Bear in mind that many are indicative of other physical and psychological states as well. Due to the popularity of drugs in our teenage society, if you spot the symptoms, the likelihood is that drug abuse is present. At the very least, abuse of drugs should be high on the list of suspected causes. Perhaps the greatest error a parent can make is to discount drugs as the cause of these symptoms because a child denies using drugs. Very few teenagers are initially honest about using drugs, and the last thing they will do is admit to using drugs to their parents. Frequent use leads to "conning," or manipulative behavior to allow the drug usage to continue.

If you have discovered or at least suspect that your child is already on drugs, you can still use material in this chapter to attempt to get her to stop. If the methods here do not work, professional treatment may be indicated. Treatment will be dealt with later, but a word of caution is advisable here. Be careful about how you choose a treatment program, as there are a variety of programs with success rates that are very different. If an inpatient program is needed, as it often is with adolescents who are resistant or unable to stop their use of drugs (both groups are psychologically dependent), a program that specifically treats this problem is indicated. You may be in an emotional state of shock and tempted to hospitalize the child anywhere. This often has disastrous effects, as the program may be excessively expensive and long-term (lasting 6 months to 3 years) and not really able to deal with your child's type of problem. An effective program is often short-term (lasting 1 to 2 months) and affordable and offers intensive therapy during the stay. See the resource list at the end of the book for information about drug programs.

It is now time to organize your preventive group and implement certain projects and rules at home. I shall assume you are dealing with children who are not using drugs, although the techniques may be helpful for the child who only recently began to use drugs.

SHARE THE INFORMATION

The education you have attained for yourself can be shared not only with other parents but also with your children, and it should be done in a friendly, nonthreatening atmosphere. For example, an open, frank discussion about the drug problem in the neighborhood, school, or community should be initiated, with the clear message that the child or children are not being accused of using drugs. Your communication should be guided along the lines of the effects drugs have on your child's age group, the strength of peer pressure pushing people into using drugs, the difficulties this causes in school and relationships with parents and friends. Let him or her understand that you know the difficulties inherent in growing up and are concerned about goals, problems, feelings of inadequacy, school problems, peer problems, and emotional life in general. Let your child know that you are always available to listen, understand, and guide him or her through these troubled times.

Perhaps the main point to emphasize is that this is a period in which teenagers can come to understand themselves better and to learn techniques to cope with problems. Since most preadolescents and adolescents have a high desire for independence, you can stress that the more capable one is in solving problems, coping with stress, and avoiding misjudgments, the more chance for real independence that person has. Examples of older kids who are dependent on drugs and therefore not independent at all are helpful, especially if your children know these older teenagers. Other parents in your group will be discussing this with their children as well.

Another step that you and the other parents should complete before the first formal meeting of the parent peer group is to make a lists of the children's friends (or children's peer groups). This should include who comes to visit, whom your child visits, who his friends are at school, and who telephones him. With a little investigation at school and in the neighborhood, you may uncover the fact that his peer group is much larger than you expected. Do as much snooping as you can to find out what really goes on in this neighborhood or school subculture, and have the other parents (the core parents) do the same.

MEETINGS OF THE PARENT PEER GROUP

Now is the time for the first meeting of the group. You have amassed literature on starting a parents' group, gathered paraphernalia, learned the frequent signs and symptoms of drug usage, found out who your children's friends are, learned more about his culture, and had some frank discussions about drugs with your children, as have the other parents.

You need to make information packets containing much of the information you have obtained. This task can be shared by the core group, and photocopies can be made. The packages usually contain a letter of introduction telling who you are, a sheet explaining the extent of the drug problem in your community, and perhaps one of the articles you have obtained on marijuana.

All the parents who have children who are acquaintances of the children of the core parent group should be invited, as well as anyone else you know who is interested. The first meeting should be held in one of the homes, and the children should be away for the evening.

This first meeting is very anxiety provoking, especially for people who are new. They have not yet read any of the literature, and the whole experience may be frightening to them. Because of this you must be well prepared. I am going to assume that there is a drug problem somewhere close to you—in your home, neighborhood, or school—or you probably would not be reading this chapter. More than likely you will have discovered that peers of your children, if not your children themselves, are involved with drugs, and some of their parents will be present.

Some of the groups attempt to diminish the anxiety by delivering information packets to the new parents before this meeting. Provide extra copies if they show an interest. Some of the new parents are very willing to provide names of other people who might be interested and may be willing to help from the start. You should follow up on all leads.

For those parents who seem hesitant, you may need to sell the idea, but let them know that you are not accusing them or their children of anything. Some parents are angry and defensive. Do not attempt to oversell. Merely let them know what you are trying to accomplish and invite their participation.

It is preferable to set the meeting up in the evening, giving advance notice and sending out flyers if needed. It is not necessary to have a large meeting initially. Radio announcements and posters can be produced to encourage more attendance as the program starts to grow.

As mentioned before, an informal atmosphere is best. Provide coffee, soft drinks, and cakes if possible, but *no alcohol*, for obvious reasons.

The person who has organized the meeting should begin by stating its purpose, discussing the research she or he has done in the community about their problem, and exhibiting the literature that has been gathered, with the announcement that copies are available. Then more specifics can be added, such as showing the paraphernalia that has been gathered at the local convenience or grocery store and mentioning the head shops and other places where children congregate. If your own child uses drugs and you have discovered it, share this information with the group and have the other core parents tell about their children's problems.

Be sure to emphasize that the meeting was called to stop any drug use and prevent further use. Let everyone know that the idea of the meetings is to organize a cooperative parent peer group to exert pressure in various areas such as home, school, community, and the legislature.

Some parents will begin to feel guilty and often will tend to deny that their children could possibly be using drugs. If you know that they *are* using drugs, you must point out the facts. Let these parents know that you are in the same situation and it is not their fault. No matter how tactful you are, you may have to deal with one or more people who will react with dismay, anger, guilt, resentment, and flat denial. You obviously have skills with people or you would not have gone this far toward organizing a potentially stressful meeting. You must use your skills to the utmost.

If you know a concerned parent who has a child with a serious drug problem, it is a good idea to have that parent present to discuss how insidiously the use started, how it escalated and progressed, and how the parent wishes that he or she had known about preventive techniques then.

The point should be made that if any of the kids are into drugs, then they all may be, and at the very least, all are highly susceptible.

At the end of the meeting, everyone is encouraged to start finding out more about their children's lives, to read the additional material, to put thought into plans of action, and to return for a second meeting soon.

The second meeting is designed to discuss what they

have found out about the use of drugs, to agree on common approaches, and to discuss proposals about areas of endeavor that the group will focus on.

Many parents have found that a unified code of behavior for their children works best. Some of these codes have lessened and even eradicated the use of drugs in certain neighborhoods. I will present a number of these parental rules.

First of all, the parents agree that their children can only have friends whose parents belong to the parent peer group and whose attitudes about drugs are not permissive. This may seem overly restrictive at first glance, but many parents will testify to the effects. It gives the parents an enormous amount of reassurance to know that the parents of their children's friends are not allowing drugs to be used in their homes. They feel more comfortable and trusting of their own children.

Second, all the parents inform their children of the parent group and its function. They tell the kids that they all agree on certain rules, especially a total prohibition of drugs and alcohol, and that they shall be enforced. The rules may vary for any particular group, and I will present some general guidelines. It should be mentioned here that the more cooperation the group has from the school the better, since much of the drug scene occurs at school.

CODE OF BEHAVIOR FOR TEENAGERS

1. SCHOOL
All children must attend school and abide by all rules and regulations. They may not congregate in areas at school where drugs are used or associate with kids who use drugs. They are not to leave school during the day. Schoolwork must be completed, and the parents will arrange a schedule to help with schoolwork if needed.
2. NONSCHOOL TIME
(a) During the school week everyone must be either at home

after school or with kids whose parents are in group. All kids stay home after supper except to go to approved events. (b) On the weekend, the following curfews must be observed:

9th grade	10:00 P.M.
10th grade	10:30 P.M.
11th grade	11:00 P.M.
12th grade	12:00 P.M.

The only exceptions are made by the parents and should be under chaperoned supervision.

3. NO DRUGS OR ALCOHOL ARE PERMISSIBLE

This is an *absolute* rule. This is an area in which the parents need to assess their function as role models. Many teenagers will feel that they are being asked to follow a double standard if the parents drink. In my opinion, the family has a better relationship if the parents are willing to give up their alcohol use as an example for their children to follow.

4. OFF-LIMIT PLACES

Head shops, rock concerts, parties at homes that are unsupervised or where drugs are known to exist, and places where large numbers of teenagers congregate such as pool halls and other local hangouts, are forbidden.

5. PARTIES

No alcohol or drugs. Parties must be small and supervised, and the adults should be visible frequently. No unknown kids are allowed. Parents should know the supervising adult's phone number and address. The party must end at the agreed-upon time. The parents should inquire about the supervision *before* the party and offer to assist.

6. TELEPHONE CALLS

Callers must identify themselves or the calls are refused. There should be no telephone calls after an agreed time.

7. ALLOWANCE

Receiving an allowance should be contingent upon completion of chores, schoolwork, and responsibilities at home.

As for younger adolescents (eighth grade and below), essentially the same rules apply, but all events must be chaperoned and children are not allowed out on weekend evenings unless they are supervised by a trusted adult. Although absolute rules against alcohol and drugs are also essential, there are other rules any group may want to enforce.

COMMUNITY PRESSURE

I mentioned earlier the importance of legislation against the sale of paraphernalia and drugs and also alluded to the effects of TV programming. This is a very serious concern to those of us involved in prevention. Perhaps the greatest damage, because of its subtlety, is done by television programming. Lately more programs are presenting drug use as a benign event. In the format of situation comedies practically nightly during prime television viewing time, scenes containing humor about marijuana, cocaine, alcohol, and other drugs are presented to millions of viewers. The cops-and-robbers shows are filled with exciting chases, schemes, and shoot-outs over drugs. Many movies made for television deal overtly with drugs or have a subplot or scenes involving drugs.

The overall effect is to change gradually the attitude of many Americans about the casual use of drugs. As the adolescent and adult viewers see humorous stories concerning people involved with drugs, played by nationally recognizable actors, they unconsciously accept that drugs are commonplace, acceptable, and fun. This obviously affects the total psychological viewpoint of young minds as well as adolescents and adults. It establishes a frame of mind that will contain less internal inhibitions to avoid drug experimentation. This is one of the reasons we are seeing children younger than eight years old beginning to try drugs. As a matter of fact, the average initial age at onset of drug use in the patients I see at my hospital, which has a large population of middle-class youth, has decreased in the last five years. In 1975 the average age at which my patients had first experimented with alcohol and/or pot was thirteen. By 1980 it had decreased to eight. Consequently they are entering the hospital at a younger age, usually twelve years old and up.

As parent groups grow, they become a large enough force in the community to influence TV programming. They can boycott products advertised by companies that sponsor these programs, send out press releases about their feelings regarding the programs and sponsors, write letters to local stations and national networks, and send letters to other parent groups enlisting their support, appear on local talk shows and write letters to the newspapers. This has been done, often with good results.

Similar techniques can be used against prodrug songs and movies. Many songs encourage drug use, and parents are often unaware of this. There are songs about marijuana, cocaine, Quaaludes, and other drugs. The titles and lyrics of the songs lead the listener to believe that she will have a fuller, better life if she uses drugs.

Again, pressure can be exerted on record companies to have them print the words to songs on album covers. If this is accomplished, the parents can decide which records are acceptable for their children. The same intense campaign against poor TV programming can be directed toward radio stations that play records that the community feels are offensive or dangerous. My personal feeling is that communities definitely have a right to establish their own standards and should do everything legally possible to ensure a healthy climate for themselves and their children. Parents should really take the time to listen to some of these lyrics. One song advises a boy who is in trouble at home to take a "714" (a Quaalude) to feel fine and walk out the door.

Movies such as *Up in Smoke* give youngsters the idea that smoking grass is the most fun possible. This is the type of event which must be off limits on the parent group list. Parents can read movie, record, and book reviews and talk to other parents about their impressions.

In addition to records, movies, and TV, clothing is another element that influences adolescents. I am speaking primarily of T-shirts, belt buckles, hats, and jewelry that promote the drug culture. T-shirts with marijuana plant designs, sayings promoting drugs, and advertisements for drug usage should be banned from home and school.

LEGISLATION

In a sense, all the foregoing could be considered a form of paraphernalia, as it concerns the promotion of drug use. Various groups are interested in enacting legislation to prohibit the sale of paraphernalia, and many have been effective. Groups in northern California, Texas, and New Jersey are actively working on paraphernalia ordinances. In Texas the group chaired by H. Ross Perot, the Texans' War on Drugs Committee, has won a major victory in the war against drugs, and I quote a memorandum from them.

> The entire Texans' War on Drugs Committee's legislative package has passed both houses of the Texas legislature. These laws will be effective September 1, 1981. The bills rewrite important sections of the state's drug laws. A description of these bills is as follows:
>
> *Drug Paraphernalia* The "Head Shop" statute will outlaw trade in and permit seizure of drug paraphernalia. It follows the Federal Model Drug Paraphernalia Act. During the committee process in the Texas House, a number of technical changes were made to this bill conforming it with the most recent court cases involving paraphernalia laws in other states. Misdemeanor penalties will apply for possession of paraphernalia, and for sale of paraphernalia to an adult. It will be a felony offense to sell drug paraphernalia to children.
>
> *Trafficking*—The new trafficking law significantly strengthens penalties across the board for dealing in

commercial quantities of illegal drugs, and requires that traffickers in large quantities actually serve substantial jail time. Individuals would be eligible for parole after serving a portion of their sentence. Conspiracy, solicitation and attempt laws are also made applicable to drug offenses. In addition, this law provides for seizure and forfeiture of the proceeds which can be proven to have come from illegal drug traffic and seizure and forfeiture of aircraft, vessels, and vehicles used to transport illegal drugs.

Delivery to Minors—The original proposal for this law required rigid mandatory minimum prison terms for persons over 21 delivering drugs to minors. As changed by the legislature, the new law significantly strengthens penalties for such deliveries, but does not apply rigid mandatory minimum sentences. The legislature lowered the age for application of the law, making any adult (18 or over) delivering illegal drugs to minors subject to the new tougher penalties.

Triplicate Prescription—Under this new law, prescriptions for Schedule II drugs (Dilaudid, Preludin, morphine, etc.) would be written in triplicate on a hard-to-duplicate, controlled paper. One copy of the prescription would go to the Department of Public Safety (DPS) for computer analysis, aiding apprehension of "professional patients" who get prescriptions for dangerous drugs from many doctors, and helping to catch "pill pushing" doctors and pharmacists as well. The "triplicate" program has been very effective in reducing diversion of prescription drugs to the illegal street market in California, Illinois, New York, and Idaho, where it is presently in effect.

Professional License Revocation—As originally proposed, this legislation would have required rigid revocation of the license of any health care professional convicted of a drug-related felony, with no chance of reinstatement, ever. As enacted, the bill constitutes a significant improvement over current law by providing a means to remove the licenses of "pill pushers" on an immediate basis. License reinstatement cannot take place unless the Licensing Board expressly determines that reinstatement is in the best interest of the public.

Glue/Paint Sniffing Proposal— In addition to the passage of these Texans' War on Drugs Committee's bills, another important anti-drug proposal was passed by the legislature. Senator Bob Vale of San Antonio introduced a bill which requires that an additive be placed in abusable glues and aerosol paints to discourage "glue sniffing" and "paint sniffing." The substance would create nausea in anyone who attempts to abuse glue or paint.

The passage of this anti-drug legislation is evidence that the people of Texas are ready for more effective drug laws. This project would not have succeeded without the grass-roots support and assistance of concerned citizens statewide.

Hopefully, these laws will give state law enforcement and narcotics officers the weapons they need to continue the on-going fight against drug abuse in Texas.

The Texans' War on Drugs is an exciting prevention program. Its scope is a grass-roots attempt to form parent prevention groups statewide. Regional coordinators arrange meetings with parents and hold seminars for the public at which prevention experts speak about current problems. This is a concept that could be adapted and used successfully anywhere. Interested people can write to the main office for information (see resources at end of book).

Individual efforts can also be effective. One woman in

New Jersey was shocked at the items she found available for sale to children and began a statewide campaign to ban the manufacture and sale of drug-related items. This campaign was backed by the over 500,000-member New Jersey PTA. Another woman was able to play an important part in the defeat of an incumbent state representative because of his support of a bill to decriminalize marijuana. She conducted her campaign for a few dollars.

Numerous others are involved in this area. It is vitally important to promote as much political action as possible. Drug sales total billions of dollars in the United States annually, and the paraphernalia spinoff sales are a multimillion-dollar industry. The manufacturers of drug paraphernalia, along with prodrug magazines and such groups as NORML (National Organization for Reform of Marijuana Laws), reportedly spend huge sums to influence legislation, and only citizens can combat this.

The Model Drug Paraphernalia Act that follows was drafted by the Drug Enforcement Administration of the Justice Department in August 1979. As of this writing nine states have passed the model law: Nebraska, New Jersey, New York, Florida, Connecticut, Delaware, Indiana, Louisiana, and Maryland.

MODEL DRUG PARAPHERNALIA ACT

ARTICLE I
(Definitions)

SECTION _____ *(insert designation of definitional section)* of the Controlled Substances Act of this State is amended by adding the following after paragraph _____ *(insert designation of last definition in section):*

( ) The term "Drug Paraphernalia" means all equipment, products and materials of any kind which are used, intended for use, or designed for use, in planting, propagating, cultivating, growing, harvesting, manufacturing, compounding, converting, producing, processing, preparing, testing, analyzing, packaging, repackaging, storing, containing, concealing, injecting, ingesting, inhaling, or otherwise introducing into the human body a controlled substance in violation of this Act (meaning the Controlled Substances Act of this State). It includes, but is not limited to:

(1) Kits used, intended for use, or designed for use in planting, propagating, cultivating, growing or harvesting of any species of plant which is a controlled substance or from which a controlled substance can be derived;

(2) Kits used, intended for use, or designed for use in manufacturing, compounding, converting, producing, processing, or preparing controlled substances;

(3) Isomerization devices used, intended for use, or designed for use in identifying, or in analyzing the strength, effectiveness or purity of controlled substances;

(4) Testing equipment used, intended for use, or designed for use in identifying, or in analyzing the strength, effectiveness or purity of controlled substances;

(5) Scales and balances used, intended for use, or designed for use in weighing or measuring controlled substances;

(6) Diluents and adulterants, such as quinine hydrochloride, mannitol, mannite, dextrose and lactose, used, intended for use, or designed for use in cutting controlled substances;

(7) Separation gins and sifters used, intended for use, or designed for use in removing twigs and seeds from, or in otherwise cleaning or refining, marijuana;

(8) Blenders, bowls, containers, spoons and mixing devices used, intended for use, or designed for use in compounding controlled substances;

(9) Capsules, ballons, envelopes and other containers used, intended for use, or designed for use in packaging small quantities of controlled substances;

(10) Containers and other objects intended for use, or designed for use in storing or concealing controlled substances;

(11) Hypodermic syringes, needles and other objects used, intended for use, or designed for use in parenterally injecting controlled substances into the human body;

(12) Objects used, intended for use, or designed for use in ingesting, inhaling, or otherwise introducing marijuana, cocaine, hashish, or hashish oil into the human body, such as:

    (a) Metal, wooden, acrylic, glass, stone, plastic, or ceramic pipes with or without screens, permanent screens, hashish heads, or punctured metal bowls;

    (b) Water pipes;

    (c) Carburetion tubes and devices;

    (d) Smoking and carburetion masks;

    (e) Roach clips: meaning objects used to hold burning material, such as a marijuana cigarette, that has become too small or too short to be held in the hand;

    (f) Miniature cocaine spoons, and cocaine vials;

    (h) Carburetor pipes;

    (i) Electric pipes;

    (j) Air-driven pipes;

    (k) Chillums;

    (l) Bongs;

    (m) Ice pipes or chillers;

In determining whether an object is drug paraphernalia, a court or other authority should consider, in addition to all other logically relevant factors, the following:

(1) Statements by an owner or by anyone in control of the object concerning its use;

(2) Prior convictions, if any, of an owner, or of anyone in control of the object, under any state or federal law relating to any controlled substance;

(3) The proximity of the object, in time and space, to a direct violation of this Act;

(4) The proximity of the object to controlled substances;

(5) The existence of any residue of controlled substances on the object;

(6) Direct or circumstantial evidence of the intent of an owner, or of anyone in control of the object, to deliver it to persons whom he knows, or should reasonably know, intend to use the object to facilitate a violation of this Act; the innocence of an owner, or of anyone in control of the object, as to a direct violation of the Act shall not prevent a finding that the object is intended for use, or designed for use as drug paraphernalia;

(7) Instructions, oral or written, provided with the object concerning its use;

(8) Descriptive materials accompanying the object which explain or depict its use;

(9) National and local advertising concerning its use;

(10) The manner in which the object is displayed for sale;

(11) Whether the owner, or anyone in control of the object, is a legitimate supplier of like or related items to the community, such as a licensed distributor or dealer of tobacco products;

(12) Direct or circumstantial evidence of the ratio of sales of object(s) to the total sales of the business enterprise;

(13) The existence and scope of legitimate uses for the object in the community;

(14) Expert testimony concerning its use.

ARTICLE II
(Offenses and Penalties)

SECTION _____ *(designation of offenses and penalties section)* of the Controlled Substances Act of this State is amended by adding the following after _____ *(designation of last substantive offense)*:

SECTION (A) *(Possession of Drug Paraphernalia)*

It is unlawful for any person to use, or to possess with intent to use, drug paraphernalia to plant, propagate, cultivate, grow, harvest, manufacture, compound, convert, produce, process, prepare, test, analyze, pack, repack, store, contain, conceal, inject, ingest, inhale, or otherwise introduce into the human body a controlled substance in violation of this Act. Any person who violates this section is guilty of a crime and upon conviction may be imprisoned for not more than _____ (length of time), fined not more than $_____, or both.

SECTION (B) *(Manufacture or Delivery of Drug Paraphernalia)*

It is unlawful for any person to deliver, possess with intent to deliver, or manufacture with intent to deliver, drug paraphernalia, knowing, or under circumstances where one reasonably should know, that it will be used to plant, propagate, cultivate, grow, harvest, manufacture, compound, convert, produce, process, prepare, test, analyze, pack, repack, store, contain, conceal, inject, ingest, inhale, or otherwise introduce into the human body a controlled substance in violation of this Act. Any person who violates this section is guilty of a crime and upon conviction may be imprisoned for not more than _____ (length of time), fined not more than $_____, or both.

SECTION (C) *(Delivery of Drug Paraphernalia to a Minor)*

Any person 18 years of age or over who violates Section (B) by delivering drug paraphernalia to a person under 18 years of age who is at least 3 years his junior is guilty of a special offense and upon conviction may be imprisoned for not more than _____ (length of time), fined not more than $_____, or both.

SECTION (D) *(Advertisement of Drug Paraphernalia)*

It is unlawful for any person to place in any newspaper, magazine, handbill, or other publication any advertisement, knowing, or under circumstances where one reasonably should know, that the purpose of the advertisement, in whole or in part, is to promote the sale of objects designed or intended for use as drug paraphernalia. Any person who violates this section is guilty of a crime and upon conviction may be imprisoned for not more than _____ (length of time), fined not more than $_____, or both.

ARTICLE III
(Civil Forfeiture)

SECTION _____ *(insert designation of civil forfeiture section)* of the Controlled Substances Act of this State is amended to provide the civil seizure and forfeiture of drug paraphernalia by adding the following after paragraph _____ *(insert designation of last category of forfeitable property)*:

( ) all drug paraphernalia as defined by Section ( ) of this Act.

ARTICLE IV
(Severability)

If any provision of the Act or the application thereof to any person or circumstance is held invalid, the invalidity does not affect other provisions or applications of the Act which can be given effect without the invalid provision or application, and to this end the provisions of this Act are severable.

INVOLVING THE WHOLE FAMILY

Some other ideas that I find helpful in preventing drug use involve participation by all family members and also impart valuable knowledge about school and communications skills. For example, a family can research specific issues in the drug field. The father agrees to research heroin, the mother reads about cocaine, and Johnny looks up everything he can find regarding medical studies on marijuana. Following the research period, each person discusses his topic and everyone learns more about numerous drugs. Often this enhances a youngster's self-esteem, tells him his studying is as important as his parents', and can also be used in school essays. Much literature is available from libraries and the government printing office. Other interesting projects are gathering newspaper articles pertaining to drug-related arrests (to clarify the enormous prevalence of drugs); articles about celebrities, sports figures, and other well-known personalities who are involved with drugs ("anyone can get involved"), researching treatment methods such as community resources, government efforts to reduce the drug supply, and hospital programs.

A friend of mine was able to convince her teenage daughter to quit using marijuana by presenting all the material she could find on marijuana research. She spent only a few minutes a night discussing the literature, and her daughter finally decided she was correct. During this period the mother became very interested in marijuana and has been a strong supporter and leader of the antidrug movement. Many parents find the scope of drug abuse not only frightening but challenging and want to do something about it. They are often creative and talented people who have prevented thousands of kids from entering the horrible world of drug dependency.

Besides the family research projects, another helpful technique called "role playing" is used extensively by psychiatrists, psychologists, and social workers in individual, group, and hospital settings. It can be useful in any family, and it has impact that reaches far beyond the issue of drugs.

Essentially the family "acts out" a particular situation that they are experiencing in various ways. For instance, let's move away from the issue of drugs and assume that there is a family disagreement about curfew time. First everyone expresses his viewpoint, and then people switch roles with each other.

If the disagreement is between the father and Sue Ellen, a fourteen-year-old, the father plays Sue Ellen and she plays the father's role. Each one takes the original viewpoint of the other and can expand the point if they wish. This method opens new issues that need to be dealt with, also, and is extremely helpful in attempting to understand others. If it is done frequently, it allows people to develop more empathy and tolerance of other viewpoints, perceptions, and needs. Needless to say, a person who develops these skills, or coping devices, will find it easier to relate with other people. Perhaps Sue Ellen will have better relationships with her peers and eventually her spouse because she can have more understanding of their unique needs. The father will develop a greater understanding of his daughter's psychological makeup, functioning, and goals.

Another exercise is learning to say no to someone who offers drugs to you. This is a technique that is extremely important, as many adolescents are passive and will accept drugs because they do not feel assertive enough to refuse. They worry excessively about hurting the other person's feelings by refusing what he has to offer. Much time in hospital and community drug programs should be devoted to practicing this, and the home is an excellent place to begin learning how to be assertive.

If any one thing could be said to be extremely important during the tumultuous years of adolescence, it would be communication. The task of adolescence is to separate from the parents psychologically, to develop more intimate relationships with peers, then to begin forming heterosexual relationships and eventually create a separate, unique personality. This is the crux of the "identity crisis," which becomes particularly noticeable when a child experiences difficulties with this phase. In the psychological moving away from the parents, communication often slows to a marked degree and is totally absent in some families.

My experience with families indicates that this is not necessarily a situation that every family must endure. Some early planning in keeping communication lines open can have great benefits. If a preadolescent feels that the environment at home is a safe place to express his personal ideas and viewpoints—and this feeling can be maintained through the following years—many problems can be avoided.

To do this may tax even the most patient of parents. You must keep in mind that understanding does not mean being overly permissive. It is more an understanding that there are different views, feelings, ideas, and thoughts that may be divergent from your own. It is not allowing someone to act on these ideas simply because he is experiencing them.

One way to keep communication flowing is to institute family discussion. If these are arranged on specific evenings, for example, every Monday and Thursday after dinner, and the schedule is adhered to, it may become the closest time the family shares. The participants must be nonjudgmental in the discussions. It is a time to share yourself with others, and no specific format should be set. In a sense it may be a family therapy session without a trained therapist present. In working with literally thousands of families with drug problems, I have found that there is almost invariably one parent if not both whom the drug user feels he cannot communicate with. During family sessions in the hospital, the whole family learns how to share feelings openly, discuss disagreements intelligently, and work out rational compromises. The main area that I feel should *not* be compromised is accepting drug use.

Often it is the teenager who, after receiving intensive therapy in the hospital, has the ability to bring the family closer to becoming a harmonious working unit. If a family can learn these skills during the child's preadolescence or childhood, they may never need a hospital treatment.

Many times parents react with unconscious hostility toward their teenagers. In some cases this is envy on the part of the parent, as those teenage years that the child is going through are lost to the parent forever. Other times it is a reversal of the conflict he had with his own parents when he was a teen. Now the tables are turned and he can finally be in control. This is usually outside of his awareness, and he may have no idea why he is irritated in the presence of his children. If he fails to exercise some thought and introspection, he may drive his child away emotionally. This may be a precipitant to drug use.

DIALOGUE

Many parents are concerned about how to discuss the issue of using drugs and/or alcohol with their children. They are correctly afraid of saying the wrong thing and consequently pushing them into experimenting with drugs. But presented in the correct way, a parent's information about what happens when someone uses drugs can be critical in the child's decision about experimentation. The important thing is the ability to communicate clearly in a manner that is nonthreatening and noncritical to the child.

The groundwork for these discussions should be done carefully. The child must become used to talking with her parents and have some respect for their opinions. This means that it is better to approach talking about drugs with a child who has already developed rapport with her parents. Since so many adolescents go through a psychological development phase of pulling away from their parents and cutting off communication, I feel it is best to approach talking about drugs prior to adolescence.

Children are very receptive to learning and are eager to it from a very early age. They can conceptualize right from wrong and ask intelligent questions almost from the time they begin to speak. My recommendation is that parents begin drug-abuse education when their children are seven or eight years of age. I have spoken to kids at this age, both individually and in school groups, about drugs and have been quite pleased at the understanding of the children, the interest they have shown, and the sophistication of the questions that have been asked.

Education must be informative, appropriate to the child's level of learning, and presented in an interesting way. This kind of education, particularly if it is combined with drug-abuse information at school, can be extremely helpful in preventing the first experimentation as well as ultimate frequent usage.

During the conversation you should be complimentary to the child and nonthreatening in your approach, and you should talk *with* the child instead of down to him. The key words need to be defined, and important points should be stressed and occasionally repeated.

An example of a dialogue with an eight- to-ten-year-old could go as follows.

DAD: Johnny, I'd like to talk to you about something you need to know about.

JOHNNY: What's that?

DAD: Drug abuse. Do you know what that is?

JOHNNY: Not really. Is that when someone takes pills?

DAD: Yes, that's part of it. But there is more than just pills. Would you like to know more about it?

JOHNNY: I guess so. But why are you telling me about it?

DAD: Because I love you, and you need to know the real facts about it to be able to know what to do if someone offers you drugs. And somebody, probably a friend, will someday ask you to get high with him.

JOHNNY: Get high? I don't know what that means.

DAD: Well, that's the word people use to describe one of the feelings when they use drugs. But being high can feel different—it depends on the person and which drug he used. Some people feel lightheaded, some feel full of energy or even relaxed. That is the mild thing that can happen—you really never know how you will feel. Other people can have a bad reaction—they feel scared, nervous, even that people will harm them or kill them—and certain drugs can kill them.

JOHNNY: But if it makes you feel that way, then why do people do it?

DAD: Because a lot of people don't realize it can happen or don't think it will happen to them. Others take drugs because they feel sad or lonely, and hope that the pills will make them feel better, or just different.

There are a lot of types of drugs—maybe you have even heard of them. There is marijuana, alcohol, "downer pills," "upper pills," drugs that make you hallucinate, and narcotics that people can get addicted to. But today I just wanted to tell you about drugs in general and why they are dangerous for people. Later we'll talk about what each type of drug can do to you.

Johnny, one of the most common reasons someone first takes drugs is that he wants to fit in with his friends, and he is also curious about what being high feels like. But many kids, especially the ones who really understand what can happen, are able to say no even when his friends are doing it.

JOHNNY: Do you think I'll be able to know what to do?

DAD: I really do. You are an intelligent boy, and once you know the facts you'll be able to make a good decision.

I mentioned wanting to fit in with friends; we call that peer pressure. A peer is someone you know, like kids at school, and most kids want to fit in with all their friends, or peers. That is the pressure—the need to do what everyone else is doing. But if you feel good about yourself, you don't have to do what all your friends do to feel okay, and the need to do what they do to get their approval is a lot less strong. Being different is sometimes hard, but in the long run it can be the best thing for you.

JOHNNY: I think I know what you mean. Like if some of the guys wanted to skip school, I might do it to be one of the fellows?

DAD: That's a real good example of peer pressure. You would do it to please them and be one of the gang. But it would be the wrong thing to do, wouldn't it?

JOHNNY: Oh, yeah. I know I'd get in trouble with the teachers and you and Mom.

DAD: Right, because you would have done the wrong thing. The right thing to do is to refuse to skip school, even if you are not being with the group. That would be a situation where you were able to overcome peer pressure.

Well, with drugs it's the same thing. But the pressure can be a lot more because at a certain age many of your friends may be using drugs, so you might think that if so many people are doing it, it can't be wrong. But just because a lot of people are doing something doesn't mean it is right, or even safe. You know it's just like cigarettes. You even told me how dangerous you learned it was at school, but millions of people still smoke—but is it right?

JOHNNY: Oh, no! You can get cancer and die! Everyone knows that.

DAD: That's my point. Even though people know it is very dangerous to smoke, many millions of people do it. Well, drugs are even more dangerous and cannot only kill you but make every day miserable for you.

JOHNNY: How do they make you miserable? You mean you feel sick all day?

DAD: Some drugs can make you feel sick, but what I mean is how they make you feel about yourself and what they do to your relationship with your family and friends.

You see, drugs can take over control of how you think about things—like how you feel about yourself, what you think about me, Mom, and Cindy. What happens is that once people start using drugs they gradually use them more and more frequently. This is often a slow thing to develop. Some kids try a drug, then try it again a few months later. But sooner or later they decide to use drugs more often, like once a week, and finally every day.

And when that happens—when people are using drugs often—they become dependent on them. They feel they have to get high. And if they don't get high they get very irritable. In other words they can't really function—they can't get through a day—without getting high. Doctors say that they are psychologically dependent—their mind tells them that they must take drugs.

Let me ask you, Johnny, do you know anyone like that? You don't have to tell me who, but have you ever seen anyone who is always getting high?

JOHNNY: Well, there is a guy on the next block. He's twelve, and the kids say he is always on drugs. They say he is is stoned—yeah, stoned—that's the word they use. I don't really know him, but he always talks kind of funny. His words kind of run together. The guys say he doesn't get along with his parents, so he gets stoned.

DAD: It sounds like his life is pretty miserable. He feels bad about himself because he fights with his parents, so he dulls that pain by taking drugs and getting high. That's another reason people get high—so that they can block out bad feelings. The problem is that the bad feelings don't go away at all—the person just avoids dealing with them for a while—they return when the drugs wear off. So he gets high again. This is what is called a cycle—the person repeats a pattern over and over again.

JOHNNY: I understand that. Buddy says this boy used to get stoned just once in a while, but then he started doing it more and more, and now it's all the time. I guess he can't stop now. Why did he let himself get that way?

DAD: People don't plan to let drugs get in control of their lives, but the drugs or alcohol often become a problem before the person realizes what has happened. Then the person has a very hard time recognizing that he has a problem. He will often do everything he can to deny that he has lost control of his own life. He will refuse help because this means admitting he has a problem. What has happened is that using drugs has become his main "coping mechanism." In other words, he gets high to cope or deal with problems, and he doesn't learn any other way to solve problems. So for him to admit he has a drug problem also means to admit that he can not deal with life's problems.

JOHNNY: How do you know all this? I never heard you mention anything about it before, but you seem to know a lot about it.

DAD: I got very concerned about drug abuse because I found out so many kids—and adults, too—were using drugs and alcohol. And your mom and I love you and Cindy, so we read about drug abuse, then we went to lectures given by doctors and ex-drug users. It really is a serious problem everywhere. But we learned that we could help you avoid the problem by teaching you what it is really about before it happened to you.

You seem to really understand it easily. Why don't we talk some more about it tomorrow.

JOHNNY: Sure—fine with me.

This conversation went well. It was nonaccusatory and informative, and it let Johnny know that his parents had expended extra energy to learn about something because they loved him and wanted his life to be happy. Consequently Johnny and his father are a little closer because of the conversation.

A very important point is that this single conversation should not be the only communication but the first in a series of informal meetings extending over a period of years. As the talks continue, all family members should be included, and other issues of family life, relationships with peers, and adolescent problems can be dealt with effectively.

If possible, it is good to tie conversations into areas that the child shows interest in. Johnny is interested in sports, and his father found a way to bring up drugs by an article that he cut out of the local newspaper. This initiated their second discussion on drugs.

DAD: Johnny, look at this article I found in the sports section. Did you know that the reports say that about half the NFL is using cocaine?

JOHNNY: What's cocaine?

DAD: It is a real dangerous drug. Do you remember earlier this year when our tight end left the team for a while? He was caught by the police with cocaine and went to a hospital for treatment. That was when the news started coming out about more and more players using drugs. Not just in football, but other professional sports too.

A lot of the players said they started doing it because other people they knew were using it. So you see peer pressure happens with adults, too, not just kids. The report says that it made them feel high, then kind of relaxed them. Some of them thought they could play better when they were more relaxed. But what happened was they lost control, the drug took over, and they started spending all their money on the drugs.

JOHNNY: But they make a lot of money. You mean they spent all that money? Just on drugs?

DAD: Johnny, drugs can get very expensive. I've been reading about cocaine. It can cost a person who uses a lot of it as much as $1000 in one day. He can spend all his savings in no time at all. I read about wealthy people who spent $50,000 to over $100,000 in a year.

JOHNNY: What does it do besides get someone high? Does it hurt their body?

DAD: That is another big problem with cocaine. It makes people use it more and more often, and it damages their bodies. Most users sniff it through their nose, and it finally destroys their nose bone, which is very painful. It can lead to their lungs collapsing, heavy sweating, and their blood vessel system can collapse, and then they die. But most users either don't know this or figure that it won't happen to them. Some people use so much that they just don't care what happens.

Another problem is that a lot of people will not use just one drug but like to mix two or more drugs together. The results can be horrible. A lot of these drugs can cause an overdose, especially if they are mixed. An overdose is when someone uses too much, and the drug can make them pass out, go into a coma, and even die.

One of the most common drugs that teenagers use is alcohol. Sooner or later you will be somewhere where kids are drinking, so I want you to really know about alcohol.

JOHNNY: I didn't know it was a drug. If it is so dangerous, why is it legal for adults to buy it? Shouldn't it be against the law?

DAD: Well, it was against the law at one time, but the law was changed. Many adults seem to be able to drink, but millions of others become alcoholics—they have their lives ruined by alcohol. Most people think that certain people develop a medical illness—alcoholism—but other people escape it. The problem is that it is impossible to know who will develop it.

But the situation for teenagers is even riskier. For some reason that isn't understood, teenagers can develop alcoholism quicker than most adults. And many adult alcoholics started their drinking when they were teenagers. Anyway, alcohol is one of the very worst drugs because it can cause very bad physical problems, you can become addicted to it, and it is cheap and legal.

JOHNNY: What does "addicted" mean?

DAD: You remember before I told you how people become dependent on a drug—where they feel they need to get high every day. That is what people call a psychological dependency. They depend on the drug because they *think* they have to have it to make it through the day. But some drugs can make a person physically addicted—he has to take it or he can go through a state called withdrawal.

That is when the body has to have the drug. If it doesn't get it, the person has bad stomach cramps, feels like throwing up, shakes, and can have seizures where his whole body shakes, and can die. And the drug that causes the worst withdrawal is alcohol.

Now, most teenagers and adults don't realize what a bad drug alcohol is because it is legal. And since a lot of parents drink, they think it is all right for their kids to drink. They would rather have them drink than use other drugs. But that isn't a very good idea. Most teenagers who use drugs also drink. And when you mix alcohol with drugs, it makes the reaction much worse.

JOHNNY: Well, what should I do if other kids are drinking or using drugs?

DAD: That's a good question, and something you need to

be prepared for. First of all, you should have certain convictions—certain values—that you decide are important for you. One of those values could be to enjoy life naturally. That means without having to use something artificial, like a drug. Another thing is to understand that if someone, like a group of kids, won't accept you because you won't do what they want you to, like getting high, then they really are not your true friends because they don't accept you for yourself.

The best thing, I believe, is to feel good enough about yourself that you can shift friends if certain people turn out to be different than you thought. There are still a lot of good kids who do not want to get high—the problem is finding out who is who.

Another thing is to keep developing interests that you enjoy to keep you occupied. Like you enjoy a lot of things—sports, reading, talking with us, camping. You need to stay interested in things and find new interests to put your energies into. A lot of kids say they get high because they were bored. Even if there are hundreds of things to do, they have no interest in them. So they give that as the reason they use drugs.

Your mother and I will always be available to do things with you—trips, tennis, camping. But more important, I want you to know that I will always make time to listen to you about anything you want to talk about. A lot of teenagers pull away from their parents. Lots of kids go through it. But if we all try to keep talking—to say whatever it is that is bothering us—we can help each other feel good and enjoy our lives together.

Okay, you get ready for dinner and I'll see you in a few minutes.

JOHNNY: Right. See you downstairs.

These conversations are examples of a way to deal with preadolescent or adolescent kids who have not used any drugs. And as many parents will testify, that is much easier than trying to talk with a kid who is already using drugs. Trying to deal with a child who is psychologically dependent on drugs can be a very, very frustrating experience for a parent and often ends up disastrously. What usually happens is that both the kid and his parents are angry and defensive, and become verbally abusive early in the discussion.

HELP IN THE SCHOOLS

The closer a parent group works with school officials and parent-teacher organizations (PTOs), the greater its success in curtailing drug abuse. Unfortunately, many PTOs function well for the younger grades but are not present in middle and senior high schools. The amount of involvement of parents in the children's school decreases until no organization for parent involvement is even present. This can be changed by the parent peer group initiating a new PTO or joining one and helping it become active. PTOs are the most effective way of communicating your needs to the school and gaining its cooperation in the battle against drugs. If parents and teachers work together, a well-rounded approach against drugs will be in force in the home and in school.

Concerned parents can be vocal and have an influence on the school curriculum. A drug education and awareness program can be started in the early grades and carried through senior high school. Some schools have found that their drug education programs were ineffective because the teachers had no specific knowledge about drugs, and the students quickly ascertained that they knew more about the problem than the teachers did. Preparation is a must for teachers, just as it is in organizing a parent peer group. Experts should be consulted to help develop the curriculum, which should comprise more than courses that contain only research on specific drugs. It must include information on the changes that people experience at all stages of development, the effects of peer pressure, the tendencies toward experimentation, the psychological and physical effects that drug use causes, open discussions between teachers and students, and presentations by experts in the field of drug abuse. These presentations should include psychiatrists, drug researchers, respected local figures, and celebrities.

Many schools use a community-based drug-abuse program (a self-help group) made up of ex-drug users to deal with their problem. I have worked closely with these groups and found them to be very effective. Many parents have their children attend these groups even though they do not have a drug problem. The reason for this is that the majority of students at a large number of schools are now involved in drugs. The straight kids are the minority group. By joining the self-help group, their social lives are enriched and they learn to share feelings openly; they belong to a peer group, and they learn techniques to resist peer pressure to use chemicals.

School personnel can also be helpful by being alert to the extent of drug use in the school and informing parents when they see a problem. Many untrained teachers just allow a stoned kid to vegetate in class, as he is less of a management problem when he is sedated by the drugs he is taking. This has been told to me numerous times by concerned parents, students, and teachers. Helping the teachers become aware of the signs and symptoms of drug use and then encouraging them to become active is of benefit to everyone. Although teachers should not be expected to function as police, they can aid the battle by keeping watch on areas where drugs are frequently used, such as bathrooms, parking lots, hideaways in the facility, and sporting and musical events at school

Another approach is to have groups of "teen advisers"—interested students who are taught skills in communication, "counseling," sharing, and the benefits of a chemical-free life. This is a quasi–drug-abuse program and is aimed more at prevention than treatment.

DRUG-ABUSE PROGRAMS

A further note should be added on the relationship of prevention and treatment. If so many millions of teenagers were not psychologically dependent if not physically addicted to drugs and in need of immediate treatment, there would be no major problem with drugs requiring future prevention. One of the most effective groups in preventing further drug abuse is the ex-drug users themselves, and many of them are present as students in school. Those that work in the drug-abuse field are primarily involved in community self-help groups, but a school can enlist them to organize a drug program exclusively for their own student body. This could be incorporated as part of the curriculum, and known drug users could be required to attend as part of their schooling. Other interested students could attend also.

The changes that can occur in any person are startling. I have seen extremely rebellious, angry, drug-using adolescents go through psychological changes that transformed them into mature, concerned adolescents who then reach out to others and help them quit, also.

These are not isolated instances; they occur frequently. This has a pyramid effect as more people change and in turn help even more teenagers quit. It is the reverse of how drug abuse spread originally.

These dramatic alterations in personalities happen because the users can relate to the ex-users' previous lifestyle, jargon, and commonality of experience. The difficulties that most adolescents have in relating to authority figures and the establishment are often averted, as these teenage counselors are so near their own age. While they may be resistant to sharing their feelings with their own parents, teachers, and professionals, the atmosphere of a self-help program may appear to be more relaxed and less anxiety provoking.

Drug-abuse prevention is a difficult, complex problem requiring the concerted efforts of concerned adults, parents, psychiatrists, schools, and teenage ex-users. Parent groups and schools need assistance, input, and advice from professionals specializing in this field, and all the encouragement they can get. My hope is that large numbers of people will become interested in this epidemic and volunteer their time and creative talents in reversing the present trend of rapidly increasing use of drugs throughout our society.

This chapter points out the difficult problems that people concerned about drug prevention face. The cause is far from hopeless, but much involvement is needed from everyone who cares about a problem that has expanded at an astonishing rate.

I encourage you to contact the groups listed at the end of the book and to actively organize parent peer groups in your community. You can be effective in saving untold hundreds, if not thousands, of lives from the grief of failing school, legal problems, interference in personal relationships, medical and psychological difficulties, overdose, and death.

4

The Treatment of Drug Abuse

I would like to begin this chapter with a few cases histories of kids who have come through a treatment program. They are typical teenagers. What they have in common is the upset that drugs have caused in their own and their family's lives.

Cindy is fourteen now. She is attractive, with a cute round face and sensitive brown eyes. She has freckles, a beautiful smile, and is miserable most of the time.

Cindy fights with her parents whenever they are together. She describes her mother as always yelling at her, her father as being cold and distant toward her. The problems started three years ago. Not very coincidentally, that is the time Cindy started getting high on pot.

Her parents say the drugs caused a change in Cindy. From being a lovable child she rapidly changed into a rebellious, argumentative adolescent. She refused to stay at home, flagrantly broke the house rules, refused any consequences, and centered her life around her drug-using peers. Her grades began to fall, but she appeared unconcerned.

Cindy's father, Bill, is a thirty-five-year-old insurance salesman. He is very angry with her, and his anger has been exhibited by his gradual pulling away from Cindy. He tells me that his relationship with Emily, his wife, has deteriorated over the last three years. They are both irritable, feel hopeless, and have almost given up on Cindy and maybe on their marriage.

Emily expresses her dissatisfaction more openly with Cindy and consequently gets into more fights with her. She feels drugs were the initial problem, but she also thinks that the entire family has endured so much dissension that the marriage may collapse. She wants Cindy out of the house and into a treatment program immediately.

After hours of counseling with Cindy, both alone and with her family, Cindy has agreed to enter the hospital treatment program—because she wants to get away from her family, not because she feels drugs are a problem. At this point she is entering treatment, albeit reluctantly, primarily to get her parents "off my case."

This family situation is typical of thousands of kids entering treatment every month. They have no initial commitment to change. They are being pressured by someone— their parents, boyfriend or girlfriend, the probation department—who knows and cares that their lives are headed downhill if some intense intervention does not take place.

So Cindy and her family will enter into an intensive treatment phase. The prognosis is uncertain at this point, but at least her parents have some new hope and some time away from Cindy to work on their relationship and possibly save a marriage of sixteen years.

Johnny is the same age as Cindy—fourteen years old. He began his treatment in a manner almost identical to Cindy. He was rebellious, angry, and failing in school. Nothing anyone said to him seemed to cause any change in his attitude or behavior.

But Johnny's parents were even more fed up than Cindy's. After repeated pleas, threats, arguments, verbal and even physical fights, Howard and Jo Anne decided to put their foot down. They decided to unite and tell Johnny he had two choices—enter treatment or leave home. And Johnny left home.

For four days and nights they worried. They had read a number of articles about drug-abuse programs, read a book entitled *Tough Love* by Pauline Neff, and decided this was the way for them to deal with their son. They anticipated that he would leave, but given his youth and immaturity, that he would not be able to make it on the streets and would return home soon.

Fortunately, they were correct. Johnny returned home, his tail between his legs. "I'll do anything you want," he said, "but don't send me away to a hospital." Howard told him, "No deal. If you want to return home, you must have treatment first. We are both completely fed up with your broken promises to change." And Howard and Jo Anne stood firm on their decision.

So Johnny entered the hospital. He was angry, sullen, and defensive—but at least he was off the streets and help was all around him. At first he refused to participate in anything, and the staff told him this was fine, but receiving privileges and being discharged were dependent on his progress. After spending two days in his room while everyone else was going to the treatment classes, he started attending. Another two weeks of going to his therapies all day, listening to other kids talk about their drug abuse, their family breakdown, and their new, happier image of themselves, and he started to open up a little. Then a little more.

As he discovered that he was not being rejected for his feelings and was even being encouraged to express more, he became more trusting of the staff and the other patients. By the end of three weeks, he was asking for the staff to have his parents come in for a family session. They did, but an argument began and Johnny left the session early. He had attempted again to split Howard and Jo Anne and to get his mother to take his side. This was a technique he had used often in the family prior to his hospitalization—sort of a divide-and-conquer attempt. But his parents had been talking with his therapist weekly during the hospitalization and were aware that this manipulation might take place. They stood united.

That night Johnny tried to break into the occupational therapy department, hoping to find some glue that he could sniff. He was caught and dropped to Level 4—the level with the least privileges. After two days of sulking he began to admit that his behavior was the cause of the consequences, and he started to take responsibility for his actions.

His family, including his younger brother and sister, continued with weekly therapy as Johnny went through his intensive hospital phase of treatment. And although disagreements and arguments persisted for a number of weeks, the change in Johnny became very evident. As his attitude and behavior changed to one of increased responsibility and caring, the family was able to let go most of their anger.

At the time of his discharge, eight weeks after he entered the hospital, Johnny had completed the program. He was highly motivated to continue in the local drug-abuse program that he had become familiar with during the hospitalization. Howard, Jo Anne and his brother and sister also agreed to attend. They also decided to continue family therapy for three more months.

Johnny has been sober now for eight months. He and his family still attend the drug-abuse program twice a week. They do not know how long they will continue, but they tell me they have their son back and they will stay involved for as long as it takes.

Bobby's case did not turn out as well as Johnny's. Bobby is seventeen and has been out of the hospital for three months. His course of treatment went differently from Johnny's, and it might be helpful to point out some of the things that occurred.

Bobby was not thrilled to enter the hospital, either. He had been using drugs for about four years, and his entire circle of friends used them also. He was referred by his probation officer, who felt he needed help with his drug abuse. He was under the jurisdiction of the probation department because of his arrest for possession of drugs and carrying a concealed weapon in his van.

His parents, particularly his father, were against treatment. His father felt that Bobby was hopeless and that all he needed to do was "be a man and pull himself up by his boot straps." His father informed my staff that he didn't believe in psychiatrists or in treatment, as he had been to a psychiatrist once and it did not do any good. He agreed to pay for Bobby's treatment as long as he did not have to be involved.

Bobby's mother, Charlotte, did come to a number of sessions. She felt that Bobby's main problem was dealing with his father, who had apparently developed a severe state of alcoholism. His father belittled him every time he was inebriated, which unfortunately was very frequent. Bobby would then leave the house and get high with his friends. This pattern had existed for the entire four years that he had been using drugs.

Charlotte made some personal gains in the treatment. She was urged to attend Al-Anon, the family support group for Alcoholics Anonymous. Although her husband kept drinking, she received an enormous amount of support from the group and was able to understand his illness and cope with it better.

Bobby did not fare as well. After some initial progress and a fairly good course of treatment, he returned home. The program strongly urged him to move out of the house, but he refused. He felt he could handle his father's drinking. No reasoning by staff or his peers was able to convince him that he was putting his sobriety in jeopardy.

After his discharge, he attended the outpatient program for about a month, staying sober during this time. His father came home quite drunk one night and began to curse Bobby because he had to pay for part of the treatment. This resulted in Bobby going out, finding some old friends, and getting high for the first time in three months. This served to spur his father on to more complaints about the money he had spent. Needless to say, the cycle began to repeat itself again.

The fact is that Bobby's chance for success would have been much greater if his father had participated in treatment or if Bobby had accepted the fact that he was returning to the same environment that was at least partly responsible for his drug abuse.

Hopefully the probation officer or his mother will be able to get him back into a short treatment course. He would probably achieve sobreity if he could be convinced to leave the environment and stay active in the community drug-abuse program.

Karen is happy now. But for years she was involved in constant arguments, ran away from home every few months, and was repeatedly arrested. She now has been sober for one and a half years, gets along with her family and friends, has her general equivalency diploma for high school, and works as a drug-abuse counselor.

Karen is nineteen. She never went through the hospital program. She joined a drug-abuse program that is open to anyone who desires to live a chemical-free life. And it worked for her.

Karen joined the program when she "hit bottom." She had been thrown out of her house, her parents refused to support her any longer, and she moved from one person's home to another's every few days. Finally her "friends," all drug users themselves, got tired of taking care of her. So at eighteen, Karen was on the streets, alone and broke.

The drug-abuse program asked her for a thirty-day commitment to work the program. She was expected to attend meetings three times weekly and to spend her days at the gathering place, located in a church. She was asked to talk to a counselor anytime she had an urge to get high. In return a member of the program would provide room and board during this time. At the end of one month, if she had stayed straight and wanted to continue in the program, she had to get a job and help pay her expenses.

Karen tried hard. She went to all the meetings, listened to what people were saying, and then began to open up and talk about herself. The more she talked, the better she felt. Her self-esteem started to improve, she felt closer to the other members, and she began to see herself in a different perspective.

Three months after she started the program, she called her parents. They were distrusting of what she told them, but finally agreed to attend the parents' meeting of the program and to meet Karen at the church.

Her parents could not believe the change. Karen

was loving, wanted them to meet all her new friends, and was obviously excited to see them. She told them all about the changes she had made and then apologized for her past behavior. Somewhat shaken, they agreed to attend the parents' meeting the next night.

Karen's parents went to the meetings for a year and became active in supporting the program. After a year of sobriety, Karen was asked to become a counselor. She attended a training program and was eventually given a satellite of her own. She now has fifty-six teenagers and fifty parents whom she counsels for drug-abuse problems.

In 1968, when I first became involved in the drug-abuse treatment field, there was a pervasive attitude in the medical field that treatment for the drug abuser was hopeless. After spending two years at a federal drug-abuse hospital and working with a "career" staff in the Public Health Service, I felt the same way. This was a government program designed to treat people who were addicted to opium or it derivatives. Most patients abused other drugs as well.

The program was expensive, unwieldy, and best known for its failures. It was termed a clinical research center, but in the two years I spent there, I observed little research. People were admitted for a one-month evaluation, followed by a six-month inpatient program utilizing the services of psychiatrists, psychologists, social workers, and doctors serving military duty. After the seven-month hospitalization, follow-up was in the "aftercare" program, a misleading term. The aftercare consisted of spot urine checks, and if "dirty urine" (a sample that showed evidence of opium use) was found, the person returned to the hospital to begin his inpatient treatment over again. If he had another positive spot urine check after this second hospitalization, he repeated the program a third time, and so an ad infinitum. The first patient I was asked to evaluate was in the hospital for his nineteenth admission. This is far from a successful program by anyone's standard.

This type of program was doomed for a number of reasons. Treatment of drug abuse cannot take place in isolation from the community. With the lack of a real aftercare program, such as an ongoing drug-abuse program, people tend to return to their old environment and their previous friends, who are undoubtedly drug-using peers. No alternative was offered to these people.

Furthermore, the staff was pessimistic about outcome and tended to use techniques that were lacking in compassion and understanding. The atmosphere was similar to a prison, with the buildings connected by underground tunnels and containing large barred doors. The only door open to the outside was located in a security office, where armed guards were present.

I would not respond positively to this type of treatment, and I doubt that you would, either. Most people would feel an acute lowering of self-esteem, anger toward the treatment staff, and a desire to achieve happiness somehow. Unfortunately, happiness for these patients was to return to heroin, as they had learned no new skills or alternatives.

From the estimates I have read and been told of, only about 2 percent stayed off drugs. That is obviously a 98 percent failure rate, and it is hard to justify the taxpayers' money being spent on this type of care.

Due to my experience at this hospital, I learned many things *not* to do when treating drug cases. Most persons in the drug world suffer from low self-esteem or low self-respect. Much of successful treatment has to do with a change in this concept of the self and cannot be achieved by a staff that does not respect and understand their patients.

In 1975 I began an inpatient program for adolescents and young adults and used a concept opposite to the one I just described. The results have been gratifying, with a high cure rate and a low recidivism rate (only 4% return to a hospital for further treatment). Some other programs have also been able to achieve success in this area; perhaps the myth of the drug user's incurability will dimish because of these results.

Parents should be aware of what hospitalization consists of, what the particular program entails, and other alternatives for treatment. The first question one must consider is whether the youngster needs to be hospitalized. My impression is that once drug usage is discovered, parents should immediately have an open discussion with the child (or spouse, etc.) who is using drugs. A number of goals should be stressed in this conversation—the cessation of *all* drug use, the dropping of peers who use drugs, and the joining of a community drug-abuse program. Many details on this phase of the problem are discussed in the chapter on prevention.

Because some drugs remain in the system for weeks to months and will affect the user's attitude until excreted, there must be a total cessation of all drugs for a period long enough to allow previous modes of thinking, perception, sensation, and in some cases reality testing to return. This abstinence is difficult to achieve even when the teenager desires to quit; it can be impossible if the effects of peer pressure are strong and is a strong reason to consider hospitalization.

The leading cause of experimentation with drugs and continuing drug usage is peer pressure. The desire of adolescents to be acceptable, part of the group, and popular has been known for many years. In many communities to be "straight," or drug free, automatically places a kid in the minority. A straight teen is a "drag" to stoned kids. They often want little to do with him while he is straight and may tease and cajole him until he joins the group by using drugs. The younger the child, the more unformed his psyche and the more susceptible he is to such pressure, as he has less skills to cope with stress, rejection, and frustration.

In addition to peer pressure, a normal phase of adolescence is to rebel against parents and authority figures in general. This is part of the overall process of forming a truly separate identity, making adolescence a difficult period for people for centuries. It is a cause of family discord, verbal and physical fights, running away, sexual promiscuity, vandalism, school problems, and drug abuse.

In the years before the 1960s, being an adolescent was difficult. With the acceptance of drugs during the 1960s and their widespread use by teenagers in the 1970s, a new element was introduced into the parent-child conflict. Teens found that they could not only rebel against parental standards but could also temporarily block out the parental strife by being stoned. That the problems returned when the drugs wore off and were likely to be worse because the parents were also angry about the use of drugs was of little consequence, as a mechanism to deal with this situation was handy—get stoned again.

This is part of the problem of getting someone to stop using drugs, even for a few days. His intentions may be admirable (or may at least seem to in a form of manipulation to get his parents "off his case"), but peer pressure is extremely powerful.

In addition to the presure exerted by the peer group, another factor that prevents kids from stopping is their degree of psychological dependency on a specific drug (or on the process of taking any drug available). This is different from physical addiction, which involves the presence of actual withdrawal symptoms upon cessation of drug use. Physical addiction indicates that the body's physiology has become increasingly needful of the continuation of a particular drug because tolerance has developed to the drug's effects. This is common with drugs such as alcohol, heroin, methadone, Dilaudid, Demerol, and the barbiturates.

Physical withdrawal can generally be treated well in a hospital setting and should always take place under medical supervision. Psychological dependency may exist in a person with physical addiction and usually does. It also frequently exists in users who have *no* physical addiction. Psychological dependency means a compulsion to use drugs to achieve a certain emotional state. This can be conscious or unconscious and is quite different from continuing to use a drug to avoid the discomfort of withdrawal.

A psychologically dependent user generally develops an attitude that the best way to cope with stress is to get high, usually on his drug of choice but also on any drug he can find. It is an "avoidance defense mechanism." In other words, the best defense against stress, anxiety, or frustration is avoiding that uncomfortable feeling by altering the state of consciousness. Being stoned is more pleasing than dealing with frustration.

If one is psychologically dependent (an extremely common situation in the teenage user), when the parents ask or insist that a child stop using drugs, the child is placed in an untenable situation. If he does stop, he has no alternate coping skills and must then face all the pressures he has been avoiding.

Those adolescents whose psychological development was further advanced when they initially used drugs may be able to rely on coping techniques from their predrug days. Those who started using drugs early or were delayed in psychological maturation often find themselves in a quandry. They have been asked to give up their only mechanism to cope with life, as they view the situation.

INTERVENTION

Once parents are reasonably sure that their child is experimenting with drugs or using them routinely, they *must* initiate a dialogue and become involved in the problem and its treatment. Many parents who don't do this become "enablers"—people who do not approve of someone's behavior, but by action or inaction subtly promote it. An enabler will often cover for the abuser's problems, such as the wife of an alcoholic who calls his office and says is is sick, or the mother of a teenager who writes him excuses from school because he is not "feeling well" when actually he is too stoned to wake up and go to school.

One approach used at this point is "intervention" or "family intervention." This technique is used by many drug- and alcohol-treatment programs. Although it is often performed with the assistance of a counselor, therapist, or psychiatrist, some methods can be used initially by a family alone.

In one kind of intervention, the rest of the family, excluding the user, compiles a list of complaints about the person. These complaints are about behavior he has exhibited while high or drunk, listing specific events, such as, "You drove the car so recklessly Monday I was afraid we would crash," or "You have skipped school four days in the last two weeks." The idea is to bring the problem out in the open in the *initial* stages of the illness.

If the adolescent person is confronted by the entire family, she may realize that she is no longer fooling anyone and agree either to try to change her behavior or to seek treatment. It really is best to consult a person trained in intervention prior to instituting this procedure to be sure you are handling it correctly. There should be no hostility or pity conveyed, and the specific behaviors that are going to be talked about should be presented clearly. Other emotional issues must be left out of the discussion or the whole thing can rapidly degenerate into just "another family fight." The earlier this intervention is begun, the better the chance of success.

I believe that the vast majority of teenage drug and alcohol users either deny their use, claim that it is much less frequent than everyone believes, or will promise to cease their usage. Few are able to quit on their own, but some are able to do it. Those who do quit without involvement in a drug-treatment program are usually those who have an extremely healthy, supportive, and communicative family. They also are usually in the very earliest stages of drug involvement, have a high level of consciousness and therefore guilt over their usage, and still have peers who are straight (not users) with whom they can begin to associate again.

Kids who are beyond this early stage are in need of treatment either in a community program or a hospital program, and the dialogue with them should be directed toward getting them into treatment as soon as possible.

To get a teenager into treatment may very well mean your being much firmer than you would usually be, saying things that seem harsh and asserting your will over someone else's. This is foreign to how we usually recommend dealing with kids, but you must understand that you are talking to a person who is really a "walking chemical" and is exercising hardly any judgment. He has no intention of changing his life-style and will not do so unless he is pressured into it in many circumstances.

The best way is to open the dialogue in a friendly manner, express how you feel about the situation, suggest what you feel must be done, and hope to enlist the youth's cooperation. If this fails, as it often does, then you will need to resort to some of the techniques evident in the dialogues. And don't give up if it fails during the first attempt. Regroup and figure out some other things to say in the second attempt, and do it again. And again and again, until the person is involved in treatment.

A typical dialogue with a teenager who has been smoking pot and drinking for a couple of years might be as follows:

DAD: Billy, your mother and I would like to talk to you.

BILLY: Yeah, what is it?

DAD: We are very concerned about your drinking and your using marijuana.

BILLY: It's my life and I can do what I want to.

MOM: Billy, we love you very much. And you have changed so much since you began using drugs. I don't think you realize how different you are now. You used to be so interesting, and fun, and, well, just nice to us. But not anymore. We want you to be as happy as you used to be.

BILLY: I'd be happy if everyone would get off my back! I'm tired of both of you telling me what I should do. I'm fifteen and I'm old enough to decide what to do.

DAD: Maybe it would help if you just heard us out for once. Usually you get angry and just leave the house. Just for once will you promise to hear me out?

BILLY: Okay, but don't think I'm going to change. I have lots of friends who do a lot more drugs than I do.

DAD: Billy, I think there is something wrong. But in the past I've always said it was because you were getting stoned. But I've been learning about these problems, and your mother and I have been discussing the situation. We feel we have a family problem—the whole family is under stress—and we all need to do something to change it.

BILLY: Oh, yeah! And what are we going to do to change it?

DAD: For starters, we are all going to visit a program tomorrow. (Notice the father didn't ask the boy to go—he said they were *all* going.) And we are going to talk about the situation and decide how to handle it. Your mother and I and your sister Jill are all going to get some help with this problem. We expect you to participate also.

BILLY: You can't tell me what to do! I don't have to go.

DAD: Billy, we've tried to talk about it before. You've told us different things—you don't use many drugs, you can control it, you'll stop—but none of it works. The situation has gone too far. And our family isn't willing to let it go on any longer. We have decided that. Nothing is going to stop us from getting this problem solved now. Nothing. You are expected to go with us, and you will go. I may sound like I'm being tough and unreasonable, but we have agreed that this is the approach we can take.

BILLY: But you can't! You can't make me go and talk!

DAD: I can, and I will. I've talked to lawyers, probation officers, and psychiatrists. You can be forced to go, but it'll take longer that way. If you give it a try willingly, it works quicker and better.

I know I'm pushing you into it, but that is okay. Most teenagers are pressured into it. I used to think it wouldn't help unless you were willing. But I found out that is not true. It'll take some time and some work, but you'll change with therapy. And we'll be changing, too. And all of us will be the better for it.

Now at this point Billy is going to make a decision. He will either go to the initial evaluation, albeit reluctantly, or he will make plans to refuse absolutely, be gone from home when it's time to leave for the appointment, or run away for a short period. A family should know that this can happen and understand that it is indicative of the behavior of a user. The drugs prevent him from seeing himself clearly, and you are essentially asking him to stop using his primary coping skill, so he is panicking at the idea. But don't give up.

Contact your lawyer, the local probation officer, and the treatment program for advice. Some programs will even send a counselor to your house to talk with your child. Try to get a lawyer or probation officer to come over; this often works.

But most of the time the teen will finally agree to go, mainly just to get you to stop nagging him about it. That's acceptable. What you are attempting to do is get her involved in professional treatment. And professionals realize they have to start with the person at whatever stage of resistance she is at. They have dealt with hundreds if not thousands of kids who are highly resistant and have a lot of experience in turning them around.

Some groups advocate an even tougher approach, and for many families it is all that can be done. Groups such as Tough Love advocate telling the teenager that he will not be allowed to continue to live at home unless he enters treatment. Many kids, sensing that they cannot really function alone on the streets, have entered treatment. Others have left home. This is a very difficult decision for parents to make, because their child may choose to leave home. It is a last-ditch effort that certain parents must make, and it definitely should not be made unless all other avenues have failed.

Another approach is to find which kids at school have had drug problems, received treatment, and are staying straight. If you can get one of these kids who knows your child to come over and talk with him, there is some chance that he will listen because he is dealing with a peer and may be less defensive than he would be with his parents.

Each family must choose the approach they will try and have alternative plans if that approach fails. I have many parents simply bring their child to my inpatient program without telling him what they are doing, since they are fearful that he will run away if they even mention treatment to him. Although I usually recommend that the issue of treatment be dealt with by the parents initially, I can readily understand why some families feel they must bring the teen to the treatment center without informing him about their plans. Many teenagers do avoid any uncomfortable situation by running away, and parents are frightened about what kind of tragedies can happen to a teenager "on the streets." They feel having to deal with their child's anger about being tricked is preferable to his leaving home with little ability to care for himself.

Once a drug-user teen runs away from home, he generally turns to friends who also use drugs. They usually are willing to put her up for a while, but this generosity seems to wear off rapidly. The other kids and their families tire of supporting someone financially and emotionally, so the teen often moves from one place to another. And the younger she is, the more difficult it is to find any employment. Usually she returns home within a few weeks, often showing some humility for "failing" on the streets. The younger and less mature the teenager, the sooner she tends to return. If this happens in your family, you are in a good position at this point to insist on treatment as a condition to returning home. The adolescent is usually desperate at this point, her self-esteem is even lower than usual, and she may feel that this is the only choice available to her. Take advantage of the opportunity and push your leverage to the maximum, as this may be your only chance to get her involved in her own treatment program.

DISCIPLINE

How do you handle discipline if your child is on drugs? Dr. Harold Voth, a psychiatrist involved in this area, feels that an adolescent using marijuana must stay completely away from the drug for at least three months. I agree with him that a period of abstinence is necessary, as marijuana accumulates in the fatty tissues of the brain and it takes some time for it to be excreted. My practice has indicated that teens can quit when they are abstinent from drugs from four to eight weeks. This varies with the individual and the amount, potency, and frequency of usage.

The only effective way to stop drug usage is by removing your child from the people who use drugs. This is difficult to do without hospitalizing her.

The teen should be spoken to frankly and the point made that the parents are *absolutely determined* to help her stop using drugs. This is essentially a battle the parents are entering into, and the enemy may be all the youngster's peers as well as the drug.

Very strict rules must be enforced immediately which will alter the entire family's schedule. The child must not be allowed to visit with friends who use drugs or where drug use is suspected. Do not trust her to be honest and responsible about this; it is unrealistic as long as the drugs are in her system, which may be a period from weeks to months. She must come home directly when school is over and be supervised by the parents. This will cause inconveniences for the family but is required for success. If this is impossible, someone reliable and trustworthy can conduct the supervision.

If the child is well supervised at home, is grounded, and you are sure she is not seeing her friends anytime after school but her attitude shows no improvement, she may still be getting high at school.

Some parents transfer the child to another school and are often surprised at how quickly she becomes involved in the drug scene at the new school. It is usually impossible to find out the true extent of drug abuse at a particular school; it is often much higher than the parents are aware. (Since a move to a new school often seems unwise, many parents remove their child from school and place her on a "home-bound" program. This works occasionally, but many schools do not have this type of program.)

The other alternative is a hospital program specializing in the treatment of adolescent drug abuse. I will go into this later in detail. The advantages of this approach are that it removes the adolescent from the community of his peers, allows the family to continue its work schedule and avoid policing functions for a while, and, most importantly, allows the teen to be away from drugs and receive intensive therapy. In addition to this, it teaches him the specific skills of turning down drug offers, learning new coping or adaptive skills, and finding alternative ways of enjoying life. It also introduces him to a community drug-abuse program that he can continue to attend after hospitalization, and this replaces the negative peer group (drug users) with a positive group (straight ex-drug users).

Dr. Voth feels that sending your child for professional outpatient therapy while the child is using drugs is a waste of time and money, and I agree. Without a complete removal from the drug world, psychotherapy is usually doomed to failure if it is done on an outpatient basis initially. On the other hand, after a person has been off drugs for a period, either through a concerted effort on the part of the parents or by hospitalization, then psychotherapy may be of great benefit. Many people receive enough therapy during a hospital treatment course and require only drug-abuse counseling or infrequent therapy to remain free from drugs.

It your child is a preteen and you are already experiencing problems in communicating, some therapy might be indicated on an individual or family basis. I feel this is an important problem that should be attended to at this point rather than waiting and very possibly experiencing the gamut of problems that adolescent rebellion can bring to a family. It is not surprising to see the number of divorces that occur after a marriage suffers through three or four years of fighting with one or more teenagers.

WHEN PROFESSIONAL TREATMENT IS NECESSARY

In my experience peer pressure and psychological dependency are the main reasons for the failure of parental attempts to stop kids from using drugs.

But there are other reasons why kids fail to stop using drugs on their own. One of the main ones is that they are not sincerely motivated to do so. They have not had enough seriously negative effects from drugs to feel that they are causing a problem, or they honestly believe that they can decrease their usage to a "social" level. Furthermore, they have had little or no experience being off drugs and involved in a drug-free peer group to realize that life has alternatives that are as enjoyable as getting high.

Kids also fail because most families have unresolved issues that go way beyond the fact that one of its members uses drugs. As a matter of fact, the adolescent is often using drugs to block the discomfort that is present because of other family issues. So it is difficult for a drug or alcohol user to stop using chemicals, because to do so means that she must then experience all the frustrations she has been trying to avoid.

Consequently, in treatment, the family problems, the drug abuse, and the personal problems each family member has must be thoroughly dealt with and resolved. If this is not done, the problems may very well return along with the drug usage. Many families are prone to focus just on the user's behavior because they then have a convenient "reason" for the family being in such distress. But the fact is that there are usually some deep-seated problems present, if for no other reason than that each person has had to adjust in his or her own way to the user's behavior. (For more detail on this, see the discussion of "Family Therapy" beginning on p. 180.)

Another reason for a person's inability to stop using drugs may be that she does not believe she actually can stop. Her sense of accomplishment is nonexistent because she considers herself a failure, and this feeling is reinforced by her family's reaction to her aberrant behavior. A great amount of treatment is directed toward improvement of this low self-esteem and faulty negative perspective of both the drug abuser and her family.

For many people, drug-using behavior is a facade or image they present to the world around them. For some teenage boys it is important to appear "macho." For some teenage girls, it is important to keep up with their peers. To quit using drugs means that they feel they are left with no identity.

Let us assume that parental efforts to assist the teenager to stop using drugs have failed. At this point treatment has to intervene or the problem will worsen and result in school and legal problems, if not eventual addiction, overdose, and possibly death.

I am going to discuss hospitalization and then community drug-abuse programs. If an extremely good community program is available in your area, with experience and a cure rate that is excellent, this should be the first avenue of approach. Most communities do not have a drug program or have one that is not of the desired standard, inappropriate for their child, or unacceptable for various reasons. In these situations hospitalization is an alternative solution.

TEN QUESTIONS TO ASK BEFORE SEEKING HELP

1. Do I have a reasonable suspicion that my child is using drugs?
2. Have I tried to talk with my youngster and been met with evasiveness and resistance?
3. Do his or her actions correspond to some of the signs and symptoms listed in this book?
4. Are his or her friends using drugs?
5. Does the drug abuse cause distress in our family?
6. What do I know about the community drug-abuse program? What do parents say who have attended it?
7. Are the counselors well trained, totally drug free, and professional?
8. What is its cure rate?
9. What other avenues are open to me?
10. Is hospitalization indicated? (If you know your child is on drugs and he or she refuses to attend a drug-abuse program, hospitalization may be the only course available.)

EVALUATING A TREATMENT PROGRAM

I will describe in detail a model program—Drug Abuse Programs of America (DAPA)—that I feel is most satisfactory, particularly for middle-class adolescents. Other programs have been developed in various parts of the country that use a similar approach. Others in the treatment field may have a different bias, and the parents must decide which route to take in their particular situation.

The various treatment modalities will be discussed and can serve as a checklist when evaluating a program. A parent should check into all aspects of a program before making a decision, as hospitalization approaches vary in their types of treatment, staff personnel, cost, and success rates.

ENVIRONMENT

Give the physical facility your attention. Is this a drug program in a general medical hospital? Is the drug program a recent addition? Is it part of a general psychiatric hospital? Is the drug program run separately from the general psychiatric program?

If the program is entirely devoted to drug-abuse treatment and is separate from general medical programs, the chances for success are greater. This is because the drug program has the full support and attention of the entire staff, from the doctors and administrators to the maintenance and housekeeping departments. There is no pressure from other disciplines to share the budget, implement inappropriate rules and regulations, and otherwise complicate the already complex administration and treatment of drug abusers. It can be done successfully in general hospitals but is definitely more difficult.

PERSONNEL

The staff should be considered carefully. Is the program run by a psychiatrist, and if so, is he or she a specialist in drug and alcohol abuse? Does the psychiatrist devote himself fully to the hospital, or is he there part-time?

These are extremely important questions. You want to be positive that the people who are treating your child are well trained. Two full-time psychiatrists should be on the staff, one involved in treatment and one involved in administration. Outpatient therapy should be kept to a minimum, as the more time that is devoted to outpatients, the less that is available for the in-house drug-abuse program.

The rest of the staff should also be evaluated. The key to success is personnel who are well trained, dedicated, and experienced. Individual therapists ("primary therapists") should have at least a master's degree. Psychologists for testing should have a Ph.D., and schoolteachers must be trained in drug abuse. It is desirable for the drug-abuse counselors to be ex-drug users who have been trained by the staff and are now experienced and professional.

COST

Length of hospitalization, cost, aftercare planning, and treatment modalities should be considered. A program can vary in length from one month to three years, and the cost will be up to eighteen times as expensive for a three-year program as it would be for a two-month program. My experience indicates that a successul program can be completed in six to eight weeks, at a relatively inexpensive cost after insurance pays its benefits. Most health-insurance policies cover drug and alcohol abuse and often pay 80 percent of the cost of hospitalization. Most private hospitals and doctors require a deposit based on the insurance benefits that are verified prior to admission and arrange a payout plan for any balance. This allows a program to be affordable to the greatest number of people.

Most programs bill for the services provided, with a patient being charged for a treatment modality each time he uses it. This causes some variation in the total cost for different individuals.

As the cost of hospitalization is continually rising, it is appropriate and important that you acquire information about the hospital and the doctor's fees prior to hospitalization so that you can have an accurate idea of the total costs and can budget correctly.

The type of hospital inpatient program I prefer involves a short-term, highly intensive therapy. The length of stay is rarely over eight to ten weeks. For a program this short to be successful, great amounts of therapy must occur in this time span. Teenagers are capable of making more immediate changes than people in most other age groups if they receive the correct kind of therapy. The results can be startling because the changes when a kid stops using drugs are dramatic. From an adolescent with a rebellious don't-give-a-damn attitude, a mature adolescent or young adult can evolve in a very short period. Partly because of the absence of chemicals in the body and partly because of psychological growth, a youngster can leave a treatment program as a responsible, caring individual.

ENTERING TREATMENT

A person referred to this type of program by family, minister, school, physician, or court initially undergoes an "evaluation period," during which a thorough examination occurs. This includes a medical history as well as physical and psychiatric evaluations by the house physician and psychiatrists, nurses' intake evaluation, and a detailed psychosocial history. The drug-abuse counselors also complete their evaluation, and then a "treatment planning conference" is scheduled. The full team meets and discusses the case, reevaluates and orients the patient, conceptualizes the goals and plan of treatment, and decides on immediate disposition.

The patient usually is involved in the treatment program

within thirty-six hours of admission and begins a full bat-
tery of psychological tests. The only reasons for not being
fully involved in the therapy phase at this time would be a
need for detoxification (drug withdrawal; approximately
10% must go through this phase before beginning therapy)
or possible underlying psychosis (less than 10% have this
problem, which may be psychological or drug induced).

During the treatment planning conference a schedule is
arranged to include all the various treatments that a patient
will receive, and a copy of the schedule is given to the
patient. The amount of planning involved in just the evaluation is an example of why a full-time staff is necessary.

Most patients receive the same forms of therapy, with
some variations, but the goals in various cases will differ
depending upon each individual's psychological state.
What I see as absolutely necessary for effective treatment
are daily individual therapy, psychiatrist's group therapy,
psychologist's group therapy, and drug-abuse counseling
(both self-help group and step-counseling). This means five
hours of therapy five days a week and is only part of the
program. These specific modalities will be dealt with individually in this chapter, but the other modalities available
will be mentioned first.

We have found that weekend therapy is an integral part
of a good program that decreases the incidence of "slip-
ping" (getting high) on a weekend pass. Consequently patients attend a three-hour group on both Saturday and
Sunday as well as an optional outside community drug-
abuse program meeting. One therapy period involves an
extended group dealing with drugs, problems with peers
and family, role playing, personal feelings and attitudes,
and training in refusing offers of drugs.

The other group is a psychodrama group and is a vid-
eotaped session. In this group members act out psychological conflicts, set up situations similar to conflicts they are
involved in, and play the roles of the persons involved.

This form of therapy was mentioned in the chapter on prevention and can also be used at home to improve understanding and communication of family members. The types of conflicts that are acted out are as numerous as the problems people have. Anxieties over dating, conversations, dealing with authority figures, turning down drug offers, problems with peers, and communicating inner feelings to others are some of the areas that patients present. During the taping a person will act the role of himself, the other person(s) in the conflict, or be an observer of others acting out the situation.

This group is often a favorite among the patients and has many positive effects. It develops more empathy, understanding, and concern for others' points of view and teaches new skills for dealing with conflictual material. Much is learned about how one appears to others when the group members actually view the tape. Repeat performances on tape polish a teen's ability to express feelings clearly and add to a growing sense of self-esteem. Also developed is a general relaxing of internal prohibitions that constrict the youth's ability to relate. This often aids in the struggle to deal directly with parental and/or marital conflicts. Many kids use drugs to avoid dealing with significant persons in their lives, as they feel ineffectual in relating to them. The confidence they learn and practice in the group becomes part of their new self-image and improves their interpersonal relationships.

Other forms of therapy that are offered are biofeedback (relaxation) training, school, physical medicine, creative activities, and ancillary services.

BIOFEEDBACK

Biofeedback is a well-known method of teaching people how to recognize anxiety, sense uncomfortable emotional states, and effectively control certain physiological functions. Patients are evaluated by a stress-management specialist, and if a high state of anxiety is present, biofeedback therapy is instituted. Patients are progressively taught total body relaxation and develop yet another coping skill to lessen tension. This is a practical technique that anyone can learn and use as an alternative to getting high to relieve frustration. It is also used in the treatment of disorders such as migraine headaches, chronic pain, anxiety states without drug abuse, and sleep difficulties.

Some of the physiologic processes that one can easily learn to control include heart rate, blood pressure, muscle tension, electroencephalic activity, palmar sweating, hand temperature, and gastric acidity. In the process of achieving self-control over physiological activity, the individual comes to discover, by direct self-observation, many of the psychological variables of mood, attention level, and tension as well as a variety of physiological and emotional sensations. This ability to induce various emotional states is consistent with what the drug abuser is attempting to do by ingesting drugs, although obviously in a manner more beneficial to functioning in society.

I doubt that biofeedback alone would have much effect as an alternative to drug use for people, but as an adjunct to other forms of treatment, it is quite helpful.

SCHOOL

The majority of teenagers who enter a hospital program have been exhibiting decreased performance in school, often to the point of quitting school entirely. Patients under sixteen who have not graduated from high school or received a Graduate Equivalency Diploma (GED) receive educational therapy.

Grades are based on attendance, effort, completion of assignments, and quality of work. Upon discharge, the patient receives a report card, and a copy is sent to his home or original school.

Although the primary goal in hospital treatment is the cessation of drug use and the exploration and resolution of the underlying emotional problems, I view the reentry into school as quite important. It is part of a total push toward remotivation in many areas—family, social, interpersonal, and educational. Many teenagers cite boredom as a chief factor in their continued drug usage. If they become interested in productive pastimes such as their own education, the need for drugs is diminished to some degree.

Prior to a child's entrance in a hospital program, parents should call the hospital school to receive information and instruction on enrollment in the school program.

PHYSICAL MEDICINE AND ACTIVITY THERAPY

Many hospitals provide staff for a variety of adjunctive treatments. These include physical exercise, cardiovascular testing, physical therapy, recreation therapy, leisure education and counseling, relaxation therapy, music and/or art therapy, dance therapy, and crafts therapy.

The various therapies are designed to complement the overall goal of the psychotherapies. They provide areas in which people can increase their self-confidence, self-awareness, physical fitness, and interpersonal relationships. They also provide new areas of interest that may further aid in decreasing boredom.

As the use of drugs increased prior to hospitalization, most adolescents and adults became less and less interested in nondrug-related activities and often did not know how to enjoy any aspect of life without drugs, including any leisure activities. Former interests are often revived and new interests kindled by these activities.

The person's participation also gives valuable information to the treatment teams for further exploration in psychotherapy.

THE ESSENTIAL THERAPIES

As noted earlier, the therapeutic modalities that I find necessary for successful treatment are individual therapy, psychiatrist's group therapy, psychologist or individual therapist group therapy, and drug-abuse counseling (self-help and step-counseling). To this list should be added family therapy (or marital therapy, if indicated) and aftercare (posthospitalization) treatment.

Each of these modalities will be discussed separately, but they all overlap as part of a comprehensive approach to treatment.

Drug abusers and alcoholics cannot be treated from the standpoint of a social norm and expected to adapt unconditionally to the demands of society, as many of their problems stem from being unable to deal with society. In particular, you cannot take away their only form of support—alcohol and/or drugs—without providing something in therapy that is able to lead them out of their distorted view of life and establish effective coping skills to handle the vicissitudes of everyday living. Furthermore, an alternative peer group that they can relate to, enjoy an ongoing social life with, and trust and confide in must be available.

Each patient is involved in a multimodality approach to attempt to break the vicious cycle of drug abuse rapidly. The different forms are all important, and it is difficult to know which one will be the key to making the initial breakthrough, as all patients relate differently.

INDIVIDUAL THERAPY

The primary therapist, or individual therapist, is assigned a small case load. It is this therapist's responsibility to have individual psychotherapy sessions with his or her entire case load daily. An individual session involves one-on-one therapy—only the therapist and patient participate. This is held five days a week and is a required part of the program. The patient is part of a team that includes the patient, individual therapist, psychiatrist, psychologist, drug-abuse counselor, nurses, stress-management specialist, creative activities and physical medicine specialist, and teacher. Although the psychiatrist is the team leader, the individual therapist is primarily responsible for the overall coordination of efforts by the team, family, patient, and aftercare agency.

Individual therapy is initially supportive and "investigative" in the sense that much history gathering, psychodynamic functioning, and rapport are being established. Further understanding of the patient's life-style, psychological functioning, parental and peer conflicts, intelligence, motivation, insight, and potential for change is being sought.

In the initial stages of therapy, attempts are made to enlist the teenagers in becoming active members of their own treatment team. This supportive phase lets kids know that all the team members are freely available to discuss problems. As trust is a key issue with many teenagers, not only drug users, an atmosphere that is relaxed and informal yet professional is desirable.

An initial breakthrough of the "defensive wall" often occurs in individual therapy. Many people, if not most, find it easier to confide personal problems, conflicts, fears, and anxieties to one person rather than to a group. As a person places trust in an individual therapist and learns that the person can be relied upon to treat his communications confidentially and without judgment, he eventually will reach beyond the therapist to other individuals, small groups, and eventually larger groups.

This defensive wall is common. It is an avoidance technique I see frequently in this population. A certain image may be projected, such as the common macho image of the adolescent male or the seductive image in some females.

Other defenses are anger, refusal to talk about anything, lying, manipulation, conning, sullenness, and various other camouflages.

The defenses usually exist to ward off feelings, as feelings are uncomfortable, and no effective techniques are known by the patient to allay the anxiety that is generated by the feelings. Much of the person's life-style operates around this dilemma. He often feels empty, frustrated, sad, or bored. Drugs are used to change the inner feelings or, more specifically, to block them. When I speak of feelings in this situation, I am referring particularly to unconscious states, those that are out of a person's awareness. They are generally sensed by the adolescent as a vague, uncomfortable state that he cannot describe.

Individual therapy helps clarify the sensations and aids the person's "being in touch" with himself and his psychological life so he can begin to develop skills to cope with discomfort rather than avoid it by escape through drugs. Many teens have begun using drugs following some form of disappointment, real or fantasied (a common event in adolescence), followed by a dramatic loss of self-esteem. What is so commonly said about drug and alcohol abusers is that they lack self-esteem. This is true, but it is only a portion of the total problem. Dr. Leon Wurmser (NIDA Research, Book 12) has presented a comprehensive description of the vicious circle of drug abuse (particularly addiction and psychological dependency) as a complex series of compromise solutions. To understand the complexity of treatment and why a specialized team is necessary for treatment, I would like to give you a review of Wurmser's theory.

According to Wurmser, following the initial disappointment (which may appear to be minor on the surface) and the resulting lowering of self-esteem (a "narcissistic crisis"), an intense sense of feeling such as rage, shame, or despair arrives. The feeling disappears, but an unbearable tension remains, and then a frantic search for excitement and relief begins, accompanied by a sense of aimlessness and restlessness.

At this point a "split" of feelings occurs, the more troublesome ones being held down (or "in"), suppressed, or disregarded; a facade, or illusion, of everything being all right emerges. Wurmser believes this split is a massive denial of inner reality.

Eventually there is a wild drive for action—a seeking of a solution to the internal, denied conflict. This action often takes the form of using drugs (and/or other acting out, such as violence). The defense is "externalization"—that is, "doing something" that is supposed to change the adolescent's life.

The next stage is one of aggression—a breaking out by transgressing boundaries, violating limits, destroying oneself, hurting and being hurt. Parents see this frequently in both subtle and overt forms. From physical fighting to breaking rules, from self-destruction by failing school to destroying relationships, the actions are unconsciously driven by aggression.

By this stage an internal despair has been established, although it is usually denied, and the conscious mind strives to feel enjoyment and excitement.

A pleasurable stage of "entitlement" is the end stage. This is an elated ego state that the adolescent feels she deserves; then she finds she cannot maintain this facade. The world of reality now looms even more exaggerated, and she begins the cycle over with an ever lower sense of self-esteem.

As you can see, the frequent user of drugs does have a low self-esteem and continually lowers it even further by repeating a cycle that she cannot break. Perhaps this clarifies why someone cannot just quit taking drugs, even though her parents so desperately want her to stop, or she may want to stop herself.

The basic moods that are experienced are disappointment, disillusionment, rage, shame, loneliness, and a panicky mixture of terror and despair.

In treatment these progressive stages must be emotionally and intellectually acknowledged, clarified, and interpreted. Newer, more effective coping skills must be learned by the teenager.

It is because of these complex, rapidly shifting psychological states that many therapeutic modalities must be utilized, and a comprehensive understanding by the therapy team is essential. It is sad for us to treat a patient who has been previously hospitalized for six months, a year, or even longer who has obviously had little active, insightful therapy.

Eventually more rapport is established with the treatment team as the patient is off drugs and better able to accept reality and view the predicament that drugs have caused in his life. He is more relaxed with this environment, more trusting of his team, and ready to make intrapsychic changes that can alter his life for the better.

At this point psychotherapy becomes more in depth—the specific psychological problems unique to the individual are approached. Although the problems are unique and each child perceptualizes them differently, there is a commonness to them. Frequent problems that patients relate are low self-image (self-esteem), unhappy family relationships, impulsivity, poor academic achievement, peer pressure, sibling and/or parental use of drugs, broken or argumentative families, lack of ambition, amotivation, difficulty dealing with authorities, lack of self-control, anxieties about heterosexual and peer relationships, and a tendency toward self-destruction. Not all these difficulties are present at once in most people, but some are usually evident.

In-depth therapy is designed to bring the overt problems to the adolescent's awareness and to clarify the relationships of these problems to underlying psychological states, as described by Wurmser.

As a teenager gains greater acceptance and understanding of his psychological (unconscious) life, he is in a position to change his perceptions, develop tolerance for his own shortcomings (and those of others), and alter his behavior. Perhaps the basic key to not needing drugs to improve self-esteem is to develop self-love and self-respect. To accomplish this is not an easy task, as most of the significant people in the person's life have been angry, disillusioned, and resentful of the child's behavior (usually secondary to his drug use).

If people around you have a low image of you, eventually you incorporate this outside feeling and it becomes part of your own self-concept. This is seen in many relationships, not only with drug users. We all know of marriages in which one of the partners is always degrading and demeaning the other one, and eventually he or she develops a depressed, worthless attitude about himself. Once this person is free of the constant belittlement and associated with someone who is supportive and loving, a new, caring, potent human emerges.

This is similarly true for the majority of drug users. If they can be motivated to spend time with an "emotional support system" (the people they depend on for support) that is loving, gives "positive strokes," and clearly sees the worth of the person and is not afraid to comment on it, they usually experience enormous changes in their internal self-concept.

The main problem is motivation. Many people are not willing to go through the struggle of looking at themselves, accepting that problems exist, and changing through psychotherapy. If all attempts at motivation fail, the cycle of drug use may be repeated over and over again. Some professionals feel that a user must hit bottom—deteriorate into such a state of despair after numerous bouts with drugs, legal charges, and school and relationship failures that he is finally ready to change.

GROUP THERAPY

The effectiveness of group therapy is widely known for drug abusers and other adolescents suffering various psychiatric disorders. I believe the chance of successful treatment is greater if a number of different groups, using a variety of psychiatric disciplines, are utilized in the treatment. For example, in some programs four different group sessions are held daily for each patient in addition to the individual therapy, as well as two group sessions on the weekend. Programs that have lesser amounts of therapy lack the continuity and intensity of those with multiple daily groups. The intensity of therapy, consistency in focusing on personal changes, and presence of different personalities, viewpoints, perspectives, experiences, and interpretations is extremely helpful. It lessens the length of hospital stay, as the patient receives a maximum amount of daily therapy rather than having the same amount of therapy spread over six months or longer.

The psychiatrist's group serves various aspects of the overall treatment. It is possible for the psychiatrist to observe firsthand the patient's relationships with peers. This enables the doctor to add his or her understanding of the patient's interpersonal relationships into the daily staff meetings.

Psychiatrists have different viewpoints about what is effective in group situations and are trained in different schools of thought. My impression is that a nondirected, psychoanalytic approach is not appropriate for the short-term groups that I conduct, although it is effective in long-standing groups conducted in outpatient group therapy.

My groups are focused primarily on what I term relationship therapy. By this I mean that the main topic for discussion is any problem in any relationship the person chooses to discuss. Most of the time the kids decide to deal with their relationships with their parents. Other relationships commonly discussed are boyfriends or girlfriends, peers, and staff. The only requirement for the group is confidentiality—the psychiatrist does not discuss the material with the kids' families. The material usually is discussed with the family by the patient in family therapy or on pass.

The ability to solve the relationship problems, or at least to begin to deal directly with the persons involved is, to some degree, a barometer of progress. As the adolescents develop more confidence and new abilities to communicate effectively and assert their viewpoints, they feel less threatened and can speak directly to others about their relationships. Once they realize that the worst that can happen is disappointment and that they will have the group and staff to turn to for support, the task ahead seems less formidable. In addition, other group members who have had similar difficulties are glad to share new techniques they have acquired and offer enormous support and encouragement.

Relationships are the substance of life; people who cannot maintain good relationships are often lonely, empty, and depressed and suffer feelings of worthlessness. If all attempts are in vain to repair relationships that are beyond hope, the teenager at least can learn new methods of relating, can establish peer relationships in the hospital, and can learn to focus his attention on his present friendships. Everyone experiences losses during life, and being able to face this tumultuous time is important.

Most teens are able to mend previously disrupted relationships with their family and friends, as the signficant people in their lives are thrilled to see them trying so hard. In many cases the family will meet the patient halfway on issues, and this is the beginning of learning the importance of compromise. Every good relationship is based on give and take, and people do not mind the interplay as long as some of their needs are met also.

Adolescents are often resilient and can deal well with changes in their lives if they have learned mature techniques to deal with frustration. This is possible to achieve in short periods if optimum growth experiences are provided.

Other groups and counseling sessions are designed to aid this process. The importance of role playing has been discussed in this and the previous chapter. Other techniques are also learned, such as sharing, assertiveness training, a twelve-step program (similar to Alcoholics Anonymous's twelve steps), self-help group, gestalt therapy, relating with others in group psychotherapy, increased understanding of their own psychological life (unconscious and conscious), and communication with parents and other authority figures.

The other group therapies, conducted by a psychologist or individual therapist, enable patients to relate with other professionals who have different personalities, methods of relating, and viewpoints. It also provides additional groups with a variety of the patients in the hospital, so there is more possibility of feedback from a greater number of peers who are struggling with similar problems. Other patients are particularly helpful with their observations and credible because they are in a similar life crisis.

One complaint that has been directed toward group therapy in general is that people become dependent on the group. This is true for long-lasting groups, such as one may see in outpatient therapy (that can meet for six months to two years), or for the "groups" in an ongoing outpatient drug-abuse program. It is much less of factor in a short-term program such as the hospital group that meets for six to eight weeks.

The complaint is that a person is substituting a dependency for drugs with a dependency for the "group" (drug-abuse program). Although this is true to some degree, it is quite obvious to anyone dealing with a drug user that being dependent on a group is highly preferable to being dependent on drugs. Furthermore, the dependency on a group is for a limited period, and the person is free to leave the

group at any time. The arguments against group involvement are certainly outweighed by the benefits of ceasing
the use of drugs or alcohol.

ASSERTIVENESS TRAINING

Assertiveness training is a method of teaching people how
to directly experience and communicate inner feelings and
giving them a way of relating that maximizes having their
needs fulfilled. There are three general ways one can relate— aggressively, assertively, or passively.

The aggressive style is one which most people respond to
defensively. It is the strong, hostile communication that
tends to distance the person toward whom it is directed. If
someone is yelling, threatening, or otherwise belittling
you, you will be less likely to attempt to understand his
viewpoint or respond to it.

The opposite style is passivity—not expressing one's
needs or feelings or doing so in such a weak manner that
they are ignored. This causes inner resentment, anger,
withdrawal, and often depression. The person feels that his
desires are unimportant, and therefore he is also. Many
persons are so passive that others are unaware that they
have any feelings at all.

The most effective method of achieving satisfaction is by
being an assertive person. This is someone who is clear
about his thoughts, articulate in expression, and unafraid to
communicate. This is the best method for clearly letting
people know how you feel and exactly what your expecta-
tions, needs, and desires are.

You will not always achieve success by being assertive, but
the chances are greatly increased. The lower a person's self-
esteem, the less likely he is to be assertive. As a teenager
increases feelings of personal self-worth through changes in
therapy, he is willing to take chances in being assertive, because if he fails he still feels that he is worthwhile.

The main stumbling block is the fear of the other person's response. This is particularly true for passive people. Many people who have dominated the passive individual are reluctant to give up the control they have achieved. They use various manipulations, such as being extremely aggressive, to keep the person in his passive position. Practice sessions in the hospital, repeated daily, of being assertive will diminish the fear of the passive individual.

FAMILY THERAPY

An enormous amount of research has been done since 1965 that falls under the term "family systems theory." A system is one in which members are dependent upon each other and together comprise a whole unit. In other words, each person in a family is part of this "family unit," and any behavior by one of the members is going to cause a reaction in the whole unit.

Although drug experimentation and abuse can exist in a family that is basically healthy, it very often occurs as part of a family "homeostasis"—a way that a family regulates or stabilizes itself. When it does exist for this reason, it is usually out of the awareness of all the members of the family unit.

An example of this homeostasis as it often relates to drug abuse is as follows. An eighteen-year-old boy desires to leave home and become independent, but subtle family pressures from his mother encourage him to stay at home. The pressure begins to mount on both sides, and he finally feels that he is in an impossible position. He takes drugs, as he has been doing for some years, but this time he takes more than usual. He is so stoned that he is arrested by the police.

Once his parents are informed, the mother uses the information to prove that she is right. Billy is too immature to leave home. Dad, who feels Billy needs to be on his own, has lost this battle, and Billy, ashamed of his arrest, returns home defeated.

The balance of the family is thus restored, and the main purpose—keeping the family together—has again been achieved.

Actually symptoms can exist for many reasons besides keeping the family intact. Many times the symptoms are designed to keep one person labeled as the sick one. Then everyone focuses on the sick member of the family, conveniently keeping all issues away from themselves.

In certain families that have been studied, some interesting relationships between the parents and the adolescent have been noted. A frequent family constellation is one in which one parent is highly involved with the drug abuser, but the other parent takes a role of being more distant or absent and very rigid and punitive in her or his ideas about the adolescent. Most often the highly protective parent is of the opposite sex of the adolescent abuser.

The adolescent abuser is in a difficult situation, which may be one of the reasons she turned to drugs. She may have learned early in life that she could keep her parents from fighting by focusing the attention upon herself, and using drugs will certainly accomplish that end.

Furthermore, many parents remember their own struggles with their parents when they were adolescents and become extremely frightened that their adolescents are going to be influenced by others, as they were. This is certainly a valid concern in these times, but this concern often causes parents to react by preventing the adolescent from individuating, or separating, from them. In many ways this can cause as many problems as giving a teenager full freedom (a practice I also strongly discourage). Allowing a teenager no freedom may cause him to rebel totally and thus end up not accepting any of the guidance he truly needs.

The task at this stage is obviously to allow the adolescent to individuate while still maintaining a healthy relationship based on mutual respect, sharing, and communication.

Some professionals feel that the drug usage appears to

allow a teen to be independent and distant but at the same time keeps him very dependent on his family for support and money. This has been termed "pseudo-individuation"—it looks like he has become independent, but he really is very dependent at this point. A number of studies have also shown that adolescent and adult abusers and addicts are very involved with their families, although they may break off seeing them completely for varying periods of times. I do not necessarily mean that it is a close, loving relationship. It may be a hostile, angry, rejecting relationship, but in either case it is an involved relationship.

Many young adult abusers will disavow this relationship, but thorough checking usually shows that they have frequent contact with at least one parent and often live near the parental home. Drug-abuse literature is filled with reports of male drug addicts, particularly heroin abusers, being very involved with their mothers.

Because of the intense relationships, no matter what their origin, it is paramount to success that the family be involved in treatment. To treat a person intensively, then return him to the same environment, in which no change has occurred, is somewhat futile. The problem will more than likely recur, and often very, very soon. Not only the parents but all members living in the household should be involved in the treatment, if possible.

Some very divergent findings have been noted in families that are at high risk for drug abuse versus the low-risk families. Before mentioning these, I want to emphasize again that drug abuse is rarely one person's fault but is best viewed as a total family problem. This really helps remove the stigma of its being someone's "fault" and stops one person from being designated as the "patient." If the family can accept it as a family problem and then really pitch in and work on it as a family, the chances for success are much greater.

High-risk families for drug abuse often have one or more

members who overlook or deny the drug-using behavior of one or more members of the family. They also may single out one person's involvement with drugs, such as a teenager, but totally ignore one parent's heavy use of alcohol or tranquilizers.

Many workers also feel that high-risk families try to sabotage, or neutralize, the effect of treatment. They often pull their drug-user out of treatment prematurely, refuse to come to family sessions, make excuses for their own inability to change, or covertly discourage the person from truly ceasing the abuse of drugs.

In many cases the user not only has this family to deal with but may be married to or going with someone who also has a drug problem. My feeling, supported by others, is that both these family or "relationship" systems must be treated for ultimate success.

It may seem incongruous and farfetched that a family that suffers so much from one member's drug abuse could actually be sabotaging his treatment, but our unconscious minds work in very mysterious, often misunderstood ways. The more open a family is at looking at how their own individual behavior may be adding to the total problem, the greater the chance for the whole family's ultimate happiness and stability.

Low-risk families show a number of common traits. Mellinger and Streit have both reported that the children often perceive more love from both parents, especially the father. I mention this characteristic first because I think fathers have an enormously important role in the overall treatment success. Men in our culture have traditionally been raised "to be men," and this has often been interpreted as being tough, strong, even devoid of tender emotions. Needless to say, a child needs acceptance from both parents, and it is often hard for some men to know how to express any emotional closeness. Perhaps this is a cause of our enormous divorce rate. The absence of expressed love for a child by a father can also be devastating for the child's feelings of self-worth.

In low-risk families the parents usually perceive their children to be close to their ideal view of them and are more apt to be available to help them with problem solving, show more ability to communicate, and seem to allow more self-expression. There is less approval of drug use, and less alcohol and drug use by the parents. Parents who do not smoke cigarettes also have a lower risk of their children using drugs.

Parents in low-risk families seem to be able to deal with their own frustrations and anxieties better, are more involved with religion, prepare their children for adult roles, and show more emphasis on family tradition, self-control, and discipline.

Most families that are high risk—and all families that already have a drug abuser—can benefit from family therapy. Most successful drug-abuse programs either have a functioning famiy therapy aspect or insist on removing the user from the system for long periods of time; some programs last three years or more. If family therapy is an integral part of the treatment, then treatment is usually much shorter and most often successful.

Family therapy is not only necessary for treatment of an abuser but is also very helpful for prevention of drug usage by other family members, especially younger siblings. It helps people become involved in the problem who might otherwise ignore it, and it helps the whole family system change, to the benefit of all concerned. Mistakes learned in raising one child need not be repeated with the other siblings.

During inpatient treatment, the family should have family therapy weekly at least. During the later stages this is often increased by my staff to two or three sessions weekly. Following hospitalization, outpatient therapy, along with a community drug-abuse program, is recommended for a period of time. This may last a few months to many months, depending on how much progress the family is making.

Family therapy does not always work. Some families are unwilling to change. It seems that some people insist on having all others in a family respond the way they want them to. These are families with the least chance for success. Those with a give-and-take, willing-to-compromise attitude seem to show the most progress.

Most families that have had a stormy relationship need a place where they can routinely ventilate their mutual frustrations, disappointments, and anger. They then need to learn how to accept each other and function as individuals within a family unit. Again, this denotes the therapist working with them individually and within the unit to admit their role in the problems, motivate them to change, and then assist them in those changes.

For families that have difficulty discussing even the most minor issues, I and the staff often help them design a "family contract" to assist them to live together after hospital discharge while ongoing family therapy takes place. These contracts are kept simple, with a minimum of rules, and are constructed by the parents and the abuser. Separate contracts can also be made between the parents and other kids and even between two or more siblings.

Generally the parents are asked what they expect from their teenager, and the teenager is asked what he wants from the parents. They all arrive at their suggestions individually, then work on the contract in two or more sessions. I encourage no more than five requests on each side. Initial privileges, allowance, and consequences are decided by the family.

A sample contract follows between Johnny C., a sixteen-year-old boy who has just completed a seven-week hospital program, and his parents.

A. Johnny agrees to:
   1 Not use any drugs or alcohol at home or away.

    2 Associate only with people in the community drug-abuse program and friends his parents are convinced are straight.

    3 Attend the drug-abuse program three times a week and family therapy weekly.

    4 Attend school daily and maintain a C+ to B− average.

    5 Complete chores at home—take out garbage, clean room two times a week, mow lawn, and wash car when requested.

B. Parents agree to:

    1 Attend parents' meeting at drug-abuse program two times a week and family therapy weekly.

    2 Provide transportation to meetings and school as well as allowance of $5 per week.

    3 Not drink alcohol at home or drink to excess away from home.

    4 Not ground Johnny without thorough discussion in family therapy.

C. Both parties agree to:

    1 No physical or verbal abuse of each other.

    2 Either party may call a "family meeting" at home to discuss any current problem.

D. Privileges:

If Johnny fulfills his terms of contract, he may stay out until 9 P.M. on weeknights, 11:30 P.M. on Fridays and Saturdays, providing he is with straight, approved friends or members of the drug-abuse program.

E. Consequences:

    1 One "slip" into drugs—grounded one month, except for drug-abuse meetings and family therapy.

    2 Two "slips"—consideration of return to hospital program.

F. Limitation of Contract:

The terms of this contract extend for eight weeks. If all terms are met by Johnny, his privileges and allowance will be increased and the contract renegotiated.

These contracts are often successful. If they begin to fail, it often provides much material for the family therapy sessions. They seem to work only if all family members find the terms acceptable and are really optimistic that the family can function under the terms of the contract.

I recommend that no one sign one of these contracts until all members feel they have a reasonable chance of meeting their obligations. Once the contract is agreed upon by everyone, it is signed by all parties and a copy is posted somewhere, for example, on the refrigerator or home bulletin board.

Another factor that is important for success is the choice of family therapist. Although some therapists may be good for a certain family, they may not be effective for yours. The best advice is to find someone who specializes in families with substance-abuse problems, then have an initial evaluation. A therapist must be able to relate well with all family members and not tend to side with either the parents or the adolescent. Many members unconsciously try to convince the therapist that their view is the correct view, thus gaining an ally in what they perceive as a struggle to prove who is right. Try to avoid this, and keep an open mind. The therapist should be nonjudgmental in her or his attempt to help the family communicate and solve problems.

SIBLINGS AND TREATMENT

Brothers and sisters of teenage drug and alcohol abusers are at a higher risk than those siblings who do not have someone using chemicals in their family. In many ways this is similar to children of drug-using or alcohol-using parents having a higher incidence of chemical abuse.

In my experience, the children who are at greater risk are those who have a sibling who is slightly older than they are who is abusing drugs. This is partially because they identify and model themselves after the older sibling. I have seen hundreds of families where *all* the siblings become involved with drugs or alcohol. In many of these families neither parent uses drugs or alcohol, and the identification is more with the oldest sibling, who is a chemical abuser.

Even if the younger children do not become involved with chemicals or have not yet become involved, it is best to include them in the treatment process. Whenever any member of a family begins to have any psychiatric disorder, such as abusing chemicals, severe depression, or behavioral problems, then each person in the family adjusts to this situation in his or her own way. And each person's way may vary significantly from the adjustment every other family member is exhibiting.

How do siblings react? This, of course, depends on the individual's personal functioning and the family patterns for dealing with stress and change. Some siblings, especially younger preadolescent kids, simply deny there is a problem but pull away from the abusing sibling. The abuser adds to this distancing by pulling away from the whole family. So in a very short period of time, the teenage abuser has moved away from his younger sibling and the rest of the family in an emotional sense.

Other siblings react with anger, hostility, and frustration. Their anger is shown overtly, or they may begin to blame the user not only for his behavior but for everything else they find discomforting. Fights and arguments are bound to follow, and the family quickly or gradually develops a pattern of frequent fighting, arguing, and general chaos.

Those siblings who are very angry but refuse to acknowledge the anger tend to suppress the feeling. This usually leads to a depressed state. People think the child is sad but do not realize that this sadness is pent-up frustration and anger that have been turned inward. This is one of the reasons I have mentioned the need for open, free-flowing communication throughout the entire family system.

Other siblings will identify with the user. They may view him as getting away with things, so they try the same technique. Or they may be afraid of his behavior and identify with him to limit their differences from him. This is a process of "identification with the aggressor." It is similar to kids mimicking the bully on the block in the hope that he will not harass them if they are similar to him.

So three classical patterns of sibling adjustment have been noted—denial, anger and blaming, and identification with the user. Obviously none of these methods is particularly healthy, and all three patterns will lead to their own problems.

Having the siblings involved in treatment is important for their own mental health, and it is helpful for treating the user also. If the user sees that all family members, not just his parents, are affected by his behavior, he has all the more reason to become drug free. Many users feel closer to and more responsible for their younger siblings than they do with their parents. So knowing that the siblings are hurt, angry, and frustrated may be helpful to the user.

Furthermore, most teenage users will be returning to this home following treatment. The younger the user, the more often this is true. So the family has to have resolved the feelings that have been generated by the user's behavior before he returns home. If these feelings have not been resolved, the user is moving back into an environment that is filled with bitter emotion, thus greatly increasing the chances that he will rapidly return to drug usage.

If he returns home and quickly senses that his parents and brothers and sisters are still resentful, angry, and blaming him, the self-esteem that has been bolstered during treatment will be eroded quickly. Although it is hard for a family to trust a user completely initially, they should ideally have come to understand that much of his behavior was because of the chemicals that were in his system. If he knows that his behavior has caused a lot of stress for the entire family but that they now understand the illness and are forgiving of at least some of the past behavior, he feels more hopeful because he is in a supportive environment.

One way that siblings as well as parents can show support is by becoming involved in the drug-abuse program themselves. This is a clear message to the user that his family is willing to expend energy on his behalf. In addition, involvement in the program increases the chances that the sibling will not develop her or his own chemical-abuse problem later. Most good community drug-abuse programs have parent groups. Siblings can participate in their own groups or in the full program that the abuser is attending.

Another reason for the whole family's involvement is that the kids very often are the ones whose perspective can give great insights into the family's psychological functioning. Parents often view problems from the same adult viewpoint, but a preadolescent or adolescent viewpoint often sees the problem differently. By looking closely at the different viewpoints, the counselor or therapist may be better able to obtain a more accurate assessment of the overall family life.

The entire family should be involved in the drug-abuse program for yet another reason. If the abuser returns to drugs, which does occur in many situations, the program becomes a support group for the rest of the family. The family does not feel so isolated and unique, as if this problem is only happening to them. Furthermore, they are taught many new techniques and methods not only to deal with the abuser but to keep functioning themselves. Many families become involved so completely in the user's behavior that they quit leading their own lives. Frequently teenagers are shocked when they find that their family is continuing to function relatively happily without their participation. I have seen this cause a number of users to reassess their often inflated ideas of controlling the family with their behavior.

Siblings who become involved in a drug-free sibling group are also developing a peer group that shares a common frustrating problem—having a brother or sister with a drug or alcohol problem. It is difficult to share this type of problem with other kids who cannot relate to it. This may be the only opportunity the sibling has to talk openly with others in his own age group about this devastating personal and family situation. It also enlightens the sibling to the enormous prevalence of the problem and shows him some specific skills he can use both to avoid drugs in his own life and to live a happy, enjoyable, chemical-free life himself.

In this area it is also helpful for friends, girlfriends and boyfriends, and even other close relatives such as grandparents to become involved. The more of the user's close friends and relatives who are involved, then the more reason the user has to be involved. It should be mentioned again that the adolescent can only quit using chemicals if she decides to do it *for herself,* not for the other member of the family. But their involvement is another impetus to change, and that is why it is so highly recommended.

DRUG-ABUSE COUNSELORS

One of the important ingredients of a successful program is the working relationship between the patient and her or his drug-abuse counselor. The counselor's group meetings are perhaps best described as counseling sessions.

The counselors in our program are always ex-drug users, and are often ex-patients of ours who have received treatment in the hospital, become active in the drug-abuse program during and after the hospital phase, found that they enjoyed counseling, and dedicated their professional lives to sharing their experience and knowledge with others in order to help them quit using drugs.

In many instances the counselor is the first to break through the "defensive wall" erected by the patient. In all cases the counselor is active in the treatment and vital to its success. He is often the first contact the teenager has with someone who is active in the community drug-abuse program. If our patients stay active in the program following hospitalization, the chances for success increase enormously.

Much of the success of any hospital program is because so many people continue to attend the community drug-abuse program. This is an area in which many hospital drug-abuse programs fail; perhaps they do not realize the enormous importance of a successful self-help group or do not have one available in their community.

From our surveys, we see that the patients who stay active in the follow-up group stay off drugs and those who drop out of the group early return to drugs. This is not a hundred percent true. There are some individuals, though few, who continue to stay drug free without the aid of a community program; there are some who join a program and continue to use drugs. Teens in the latter group usually drop out of the program early or when their drug use is discovered.

During the hospitalization phase, the counselor has many roles. He leads "self-help groups," "step-counseling" sessions, has individual counseling, and is a liaison with the community drug program.

"Step-counseling" is a daily session for patients that teaches a twelve-step program, similar to AA's twelve steps, to enable participants to stay off drugs. It offers a framework to depend on for assistance in handling daily decisions. An important and necessary step is admitting that chemicals have caused at least part of an adolescent's life to become unmanageable. Other steps have to do with avoiding people who use drugs or cause constant emotional stress, making amends to people the user has harmed, and believing in a "higher power" as he or she understands it (a nondenominational spiritual growth).

These are the twelve steps drawn up by the Palmer Drug Abuse Program, a group that I find most effective.

1. We admitted that mind-changing chemicals had caused at least part of our lives to become unmanageable.
2. We found it necessary to "Stick with Winners" in order for us to grow.
3. We realized that a Higher Power, expressed through our love for each other, can help restore us to sanity.
4. We made a decision to turn our will and our lives over to the care of God, as we understand him.
5. We made a searching and fearless moral inventory of ourselves.
6. We admitted to God, to ourselves, and to another human being the exact nature of our wrongs.
7. We became willing to allow our Higher Power, through the love of the group, to help us change.
8. We made a list of all persons we had harmed and became willing to make amends to them all.
9. We made direct amends to such people, whenever possible, except when to do so would injure them, others, or ourselves.
10. We have continued to look at ourselves and when wrong, promptly admitted it.
11. We have sought through prayer and meditation to improve our conscious contact with our Higher Power, that we have chosen to call God, praying only for knowledge of His will for us and courage to carry that out.
12. We, having had a spiritual awakening as a result of these steps, tried to carry our love and understanding to others, and to practice these principles in our daily lives.

These steps have proved to be of much help to kids who are trying to end their drug dependency. Many of us feel the abusers of drugs are similar in a lot of ways to alcoholics. Even though they may use drugs sparingly, they invariably increase their dosage and again become dependent.

Only an approach of total abstinence from all drugs, including alcohol, seems to be effective for the vast majority of drug abusers. The steps, counseling, and therapy of the hospital and community programs are designed to assist people in avoiding *any* use of drugs.

Self-help groups also teach various aids to help an adolescent maintain effective functioning. Responsibility, honesty, sharing, expressing feelings, helping oneself by helping others, and other valuable topics are discussed.

I cannot begin to stress how important well-trained, effective counselors are for overall success. The hospital treatment is the beginning phase, and the continuation of growth in a community drug-abuse program is the final phase of treatment.

The understanding, empathy, and integrity of the counselor are obviously of paramount importance. If the counselor is plagued by indecision, indifference, and intolerance, the patient develops little confidence. Professionals on the East Coast have related to me numerous instances of "drug-abuse counselors" smoking marijuana with new members and telling the parents to relax their attitude about drugs and all will be fine. This is an absurdity, and the communities should not allow this situation to exist.

A counselor does not have all the answers, and cannot guarantee success, but should be someone who is willing to put forth full effort to combat drug abuse, not promote it.

COMMUNITY DRUG-ABUSE PROGRAMS

A dearth of effective self-help groups in most regions accounts for the difficulties communities have both in preventing drug dependency and in treating the users. An alternative social option must be present or the users feel deprived of social contact with their peers. If they continue with their present peers, they continue using drugs. If they try to relate to "straights," they find that they do not understand the ex-users' life experiences.

The option is to have a new peer group that is composed of ex-users who have the similar goal of quitting their drug habit. By sharing experiences, anxieties, parental problems, school difficulties, and value systems, a more mature, realistic approach to lessening the bonds of drug dependency gradually develops.

There is much role modeling in these self-help groups. Newer members see the more advanced participants functioning socially and psychologically without reverting to drugs. This increases the credibility of the effectiveness of the drug program, especially when the novice member has used drugs with an older member prior to joining the program. In instances in which no prior contact was established, the counselors relate their own struggles with drugs and give direct, valuable advice to aid the newcomers.

The technique of direct confrontation is often used and is in general more effective coming from an ex-drug abuser than from a professional or a parent. Direct confrontation is very assertive questioning about one's behavior, attitude, drug use, or other pertinent actions. Since active users of drugs are not particularly trustworthy, this tough line of questioning is necessary to defuse the manipulation, conning, and falsification that are inherent in the drug scene.

Counselors are well versed in this behavior, as they have used it themselves, often for years, when they were dependent on drugs. "You can't con a con" is a favorite expression of many counselors; they have had more experience on the streets manipulating people than the newcomer to the drug group. They have developed an intuitive feeling for others' evasiveness, and they use their understanding to help develop honesty and responsibility in someone who may relate only by deceiving others.

Most drug-dependent kids I have treated were not always manipulative. They developed the strategy as a coping mechanism to avoid detection of their drug usage and subsequent behavior. If they practice manipulation extensively, this gradually replaces earlier learned adaptive techniques and may exclude honesty entirely. One patient became habituated to lying to such a degree that he would give an incorrect answer if asked the time of day.

Parents often become aware of this behavior and feel resentful and distrustful of their offspring. An important ingredient for a successful community program is the active involvement of the parents of the abuser. When a teenager sees that her parents are willing to devote their time and energies to participating, sharing, and attending the program, she may change her attitude that her parents do not care.

The drug program I usually refer discharged hospital patients to has arranged a unique program for servicing its members, whom they divide into four groups—a younger group (for children up to 16 years old), an older group (for 17 to 25 years old), an "others" group (for those 25 and older), and a parents group. The groups meet in churches that donate space. Group satellites reach all parts of the city. This enables anyone to easily attend a group appropriate to his age. Meetings vary with the groups, usually occurring two to three times weekly. Anyone desiring to attend additional meetings need only visit another satellite on nights that his group does not meet.

Weekends are filled with group meetings, outings, dances, sports events, and money-raising functions to support the program. Some are exclusive to certain age groups or satellites; others are all-inclusive.

The parents group should be mentioned in more detail, as it is extremely imporant. In general, the more active the parents are in the treatment process, the better the results. Parents are taught methods to deal with their children's drug usage at home, assist them in continuing to receive counseling, and encourage them in various ways. An equally important aspect of the parents' education is learning how to continue to live their own lives, whether their teenagers ultimately give up drugs or continue to use them. Many parents are so involved in the problem at home that it prevents them from having any life outside the home. By sharing their experiences with other parents, they regain control of their lives and come to feel that all is not hopeless. I know many parents who have continued to be active in drug-abuse programs in spite of the fact that their teenagers have dropped out.

Parent groups in a drug-abuse program have some similarity to the parent peer groups discussed in the chapter on prevention, but they differ in that they have the aid of the drug-abuse counselors in dealing with their children. Many parents belong to both groups and are active in both prevention and treatment.

The importance of community drug-abuse programs cannot be overly stressed. It is essential that adolescents have "positive peers" who are ex-users to relate with initially when they complete their hospital treatment, as the overall course of treatment must include a drug-free environment in the home community. Counselors are usually extremely caring, sensitive people who are of inestimable assistance to families dealing with the multiple problems caused by drug usage.

Drug or alcohol abuse can occur in any family, regardless of religion, family composition, socioeconomic status, or geographical area. Given the pandemic substance abuse in the United States, parents owe it to their children to become familiar with the preventive techniques described here, as well as those offered by groups listed in the Resources section at the end of this book. Knowledge of the signs and symptoms of drug abuse, treatment programs, local parents groups, and available literature can lead to early detection and successful treatment of the chemically dependent adolescent.

You should not be timid or unsuspecting if you notice changes in the behavior or attitude in your child. These changes in an adolescent are often due to the physical or psychological effects of chemicals. If drug abuse *is* the problem, you will need all the patience, knowledge, and professional assistance you can find. It is better to be thought of as an overly suspicious parent than to lose your child to a lifetime of drug dependence.

Drug Glossary

A

Acapulco gold—a very potent strain of marijuana that comes from an area near Acapulco, Mexico.

acid—slang name for LSD (d-lysergic acid diethylamide).

acid freak—a person showing strange and bizarre behavior because of the use of LSD.

acid head—a heavy user of LSD.

addiction—controversial definitions. In this book it means a state in which a person is physically in need of a drug(s). If he does not get this drug or one with a similar pharmaceutical effect, he will experience a withdrawal state from the drug. "Addiction" should not be confused with "dependency," which means a psychological need for the drug, with or without physical addiction.

A-head—frequent user of amphetamines.

alcohol—ethanol, ethyl chloride. A central nervous system depressant that can be used socially. Greater amounts can lead to inebriation, a drunken, intoxicated state, and eventual passing out and death. A person can be psychologically dependent and/or physically addicted to alcohol. Withdrawal is serious and often fatal if not medically supervised.

allobarbital—an intermediate-acting barbiturate.

alphaprodine—a synthetic opiate used for the relief of pain.

Amanita muscaria—also known as fly agaric. A type of mushroom that has psychedelic qualities. Can cause aggression and paranoia. May result in circulatory failure and death.

amobarbital—intermediate-acting barbiturate. Brand names include Amytal, Tuinal.

amphetamines—These drugs produce a stimulant effect on the user, who will exhibit increased energy and feelings of euphoria. Psychological dependency is frequent, physical addiction debatable. Sold as Benzedrine, Biphetamine, Dexedrine, Dexamyl, Eskatrol, Methadrine, Desoxyn, and Ambar, to name a few.

amyl nitrite—"poppers." Dilates blood vessels. Used to stimulate sexual experience when inhaled. Short-acting. Irritability is a side effect. Slang name—"amys."

analgesic—drug that produces pain relief.

anesthetics—drugs, often administered as gases or intravenously, used in surgery for sedation. Nitrous oxide is commonly abused.

angel dust—slang for PCP (phencyclidine).

antihistamines—drugs used for control of allergic symptoms. Abused by combining with other drugs, such as codeine and alcohol. Can be fatal if overdosed.

ataraxic drugs—tranquilizer drugs.

B

bad trip—unpleasant experience on a drug, such as a paranoid state or psychosis.

bag—measure for sale of some drugs, such as heroin. A heroin bag usually contains about five grains of diluted heroin. Prices vary according to supply and potency.

bang—injection of narcotics.

barbiturates—drugs that depress the central nervous system and produce sedation. A person can be both psychologically dependent on and physically addicted to barbiturates. Medically used as sleeping pills, anticonvulsants. Death can occur, especially when taken in combination with other drugs, such as alcohol. Common brand names include Alurate, Luminal, Amytal, Tuinal, Nembutal, and Seconal.

beat—street term meaning to cheat someone.

belladonna—slang: beautiful lady. From the plant family. Can easily be fatal if overdosed. Has medical uses as a muscle relaxant.

benzene—an inhalant that is often fatal due to its high toxicity. Causes blood diseases as well.

benzodiazepine—minor tranquilizer. Common ones are Valium, Librium, Dalmane. Can produce dependency and addiction.

bhang—slang for marijuana. Used in India mainly.

big C—cocaine.

big chief—mescaline.

big D—LSD.

big H—heroin.

black beauties—Biphetamine, an amphetamine.

black mollies—Biphetamine, an amphetamine.

black Russian—hashish.

blow—to smoke marijuana, to sniff heroin.

blow your mind—to drastically alter a person's state of mind or cause great surprise.

blues—depressed; or cyanotic, blue color from respiratory depression from a drug.

bombed out—high from a drug.

boost—to steal.

brick—can be a pressed block of marijuana or opium.

bring down—come off a drug, arrest, depression.

brown—brown-colored heroin, usually Mexican in origin.

brownies—Dexedrine capsules. Also a favorite of marijuana smokers is to bake marijuana into brownies.

bummer or bum trip—bad experience on a drug.

burn—cheat, steal, or otherwise "rip off" someone.

burn out—to quit drugs or tire of the drug scene. Also someone whose mind has been "burned out."

bust—raid or arrest for illegal possession, or arrest on another charge.

buzz—get a slightly high from a drug.

C

"C"—cocaine.

cactus—mescaline or peyote.

candy—drugs.

candyman—drug supplier.

cannabis—marijuana and its derivatives.

carry—to have drugs in one's possession.

changes—unexpected events, such as a jail term, lack of drugs.

charge—the legal charge against someone. Also the rush sensation produced by a drug.

chasing the dragon—a particular way of inhaling heroin.

chemical—term used for substances that are abused. Can refer to any drug that is in the system.

Chinese white—a very pure white heroin.

chipping—to be using drugs in an irregular, infrequent manner in a quantity small enough not to become addicted.

chlorpromazine—Thorazine, a major antipsychotic tranquilizer used in the treatment of schizophrenia and other psychotic states, such as a drug-induced psychosis.

clean—drug free, or not having drugs in one's possession. Also free from any suspicion.

cleaning fluids—commonly abused household inhalants. See section on inhalants.

coca—the bush that has leaves that contain the alkaloid that cocaine is derived from.

cocaine—see section on cocaine. A powerful psychological and physical stimulant.

codeine—a derivative of opium. Medically used as a cough suppressant. Mildly addictive. Addiction to it was more common in the past.

coke—cocaine.

cold—to stop using drugs without medical detoxification, as in "cold turkey."

Colombian—a high-potency marijuana.

come down—the normal state one functions in after the effects of a drug wear off.

connect—to buy drugs.

connection—someone from whom you can buy your drugs.

contact—the person who can supply drugs.

cop—buy drugs.

crank—amphetamines.

crash—come off hard from a drug. Also to sleep.

cross-tolerance—a built-up tolerance to a drug or to other drugs with similar pharmaceutical effects.

crystal—certain amphetamines that are particularly potent.

cube—a sugar cube laced with LSD.

cut—dilute a drug by mixing another substance with it.

D

"D"—Dilaudids, Doriden.

Darvon—a pain reliever that is frequently prescribed.

deal—sell drugs.

deliriants—inhalants that cause a state of delirium in the user.

Demerol—a synthetic opiate used for pain relief. Has addicting potential when used excessively.

dependence—controversial definitions. In this book it

means psychological dependence on a drug or the process of using any drugs.

Desoxyn—type of strong amphetamine, methamphetamine that is often injected.

Dexamyl—a drug containing both dextroamphetamine and amobarbital that is prescribed for weight control but is often abused.

Dexedrine—an amphetamine. Slang: dexies.

Dilaudid—a synthetic opiate that contains hydromorphone hydrochloride, it is very addicting when injected. Rapidly becoming a favorite drug. Hard withdrawal.

Dolophine—a synthetic opiate. Stronger than morphine. Addicting. Used as methadone as a substitute for other opium-derived drugs such as heroin.

dope—any drug.

Doriden—a sedative drug similar to a barbiturate with addicting potential; overdose is frequent. Death can result from overdose.

downer—a sedating drug, such as barbiturates or major tranquilizers.

dried out—having gone through a withdrawal program for drugs or alcohol.

druggies—people who use and experiment freely with drugs.

duby—marijuana.

dusting—sprinkling one substance on another, such as dusting marijuana with PCP or heroin.

E

elephant—PCP.

Equanil—minor tranquilizer that can be addicting.

ethanol—alcohol.

ether—a depressant anesthetic. Rarely abused now.

ethyl alcohol—alcohol.

F

factory—place where illicit drugs are prepared for sale.

feds—narcotics officers.

fiend—someone who uses drugs as much as he can.

fix—to inject narcotics.

flake—cocaine.

flip out—become psychotic or irrational.

flush (flash)—onset of pleasurable feelings from the initial effects of a drug.

fours—Tylenol #4 (with codeine).

freak—have a bad reaction to a drug, become psychotic. One who prefers a certain drug of choice, as in "acid freak."

freak out—panic or become psychotic from a drug.

fruit salad (fruit punch)—mixing a number of drugs together. May have alcohol added to make it into a punch.

fuzz—police or narcotics agents.

G

gasoline—volatile inhalant that can be sniffed to produce a high.

get off—feel a drug's effects.

glue sniffing—inhaling model glue to produce a euphoric state.

glutethimide—Doriden. Similar to barbiturates. Can be addicting. Overdose potential.

gold—Acapulco gold (strong marijuana).

goofball—barbiturate. Silly person.

guide—the person who helps another through a drug experience, particularly a hallucinogenic experience.

gunga (ganja)—marijuana.

H

"H"—heroin.

habit—physical addiction to a drug. Usually denotes heroin addiction.

hallucinogen—a drug that produces hallucinations, such as LSD, peyote, mescaline.

hard drugs—drugs that have addictive qualities.

Harrison Narcotics Act—The United States first narcotics law.

hash—hashish.

hashish—related to but stronger than marijuana.

hash oil—also stronger than marijuana.

head—heavy user of drugs. Also denotes a particular type of user, such as "pot head."

hearts—amphetamines.

heaven—cocaine.

heavenly blue—morning glory seeds, a hallucinogenic drug.

hemp—marijuana.

heroin—highly addictive derivative of the opium class.

high—the state of mind that a drug causes.

hippie—term from the 1960s for large number of people who used drugs, dressed shabbily, were involved in mysticism, nonaggression, and withdrawal from the mainstream of society.

hit—ingestion of a drug by any route of administration.

hold—possess drugs.

hooked—addicted.

hooking—prostitution, often to obtain money for drugs.

horse—heroin.

huffer—one who uses inhalants.

hustling—illicitly obtaining money for drugs.

I

Indian hemp—*cannabis sativa*.

inhalants—volatile substances that are inhaled to get high. Can be gaseous or vaporous anesthetics, amyl nitrite, volatile hydrocarbons.

J

"J"—marijuana.

jag—extended period of using a drug.

joint—marijuana cigarette.

juice—alcohol.

junk—usually heroin, but can be any drug.

junkie—usually a heroin addict. Occasionally means some-one who uses any drug heavily.

K

kick—break the drug habit.

kickback—relapse back into drug usage.

kicks—pleasure for pleasure's sake.

killer—strong drug.

killer weed—strong marijuana, or marijuana sprinkled with PCP.

kilo—kilogram (2.2 pounds). Large measures of drugs are in kilos.

kit—equipment used to inject drugs.

L

"L"—LSD.

lady snow—cocaine.

laudanum—a concoction of alcohol and opium. Not used currently. Caused addiction in unsuspecting people in nineteenth century.

laughing gas—nitrous oxide.

leapers—amphetamines.

legal high—drugs that can produce a euphoric state but are not illegal. Nitrites (except amyl nitrite), dill, nutmeg, and others.

Librium—minor tranquilizer. Can be habit forming.

lid—measure for a bag of marijuana, usually containing about one ounce.

loaded—high on drugs or alcohol.

LSD, LSD-25—hallucinogenic drug.

luding, luding out—using Quaaludes (methaqualone).

M

"M"—morphine.

magic mushrooms—psychedelic mushrooms.

mainline—to inject a drug directly into the vein, such as with heroin.

maintenance therapy—giving enough of a drug to prevent withdrawal symptoms, such as in methadone maintenance programs for heroin addicts.

major tranquilizer—drugs that have antipsychotic qualities. Used in psychiatric illnesses. Common ones are Thorazine, Stelazine, Mellaril, Prolixin, Haldol, and Navane.

marijuana—derivative of *Cannabis sativa*.

matchbox—measurement for a small amount of marijuana.

mescalin—the hallucinogen in the peyote plant.

methadone—synthetic opiate used in place of heroin in methadone maintenance programs.

methamphetamine—the most potent class of amphetamines. Methedrine and Desoxyn are in this class.

methaqualone—Mandrax, Quaalude. Nonbarbiturate, but similar to barbiturates. Very commonly abused now.

M.J.—marijuana.

monkey—the addiction.

morphine—derivative of opium. Addicting.

N

narc—narcotics officer.

narcotic—drug that relieves pain and is addicting.

needle—hypodermic needle used for drug injection.

nickel—$5 bag of small amount of heroin or marijuana.

nitrous oxide—anesthetic that is inhaled. Called laughing gas. Chemical composition of N_2O.

Noctec—chloral hydrate. A sedative-hypnotic used for sleep.

nod—the drowsiness or sleep produced by a drug.

nutmeg—a large enough dosage can produce a high in the user, including hallucinations.

O

"O"—opium.

O.D.—overdose.

on the needle—using narcotics intravenously.

opiate—a subclassification of the narcotics (opium, opiates, opiods). Opiates are the alkaloids of opium (morphine, codeine) and their synthetic derivatives.

opiods—synthetic drugs that produce the same effects as the opiates.

opium—the narcotic from which all the other narcotics are derived.

overdose—the state produced when an excess of a drug is taken into the body. Result is often coma, respiratory and circulatory depression, and subsequent death.

P

Panama gold, red—potent marijuana grown in Panama.

panic—a psychological state produced by certain drugs, such as LSD. Also the situation addicts find them selves in when their supply is unusually low.

papers—usually means cigarette papers for rolling joints of marijuana.

paraldehyde—previously used sedative drug prior to the discovery of barbiturates.

paranoia—a persecutory state that can be part of a psychological illness or a secondary drug effect.

PCP—phencyclidine.

pep pills—amphetamines, stimulants.

peyote—hallucinogenic cactus.

phenyclidine—PCP, angel dust, elephant tranquilizer.

Placidyl—nonbarbiturate sleeping pill. Can cause dependency and addiction. Dangerous when overdosed.

poly-drug abuse—the use of many different drugs, either taken individually at different times or simultaneously.

poppers—glass capsules of amyl nitrite that are "popped" (broken) open and sniffed. Slang name for amyl nitrite.

pot—marijuana.

potentiate—to increase the effects, as when one drug potentiates the effects of a second drug when they are taken together.

psychedelic—supposedly mind expanding. A drug that causes a state of altered perceptions and sensations, usually a hallucinogenic drug.

psychological (psychic) dependence—the psychological desire for a drug. It can exist without physical addiction or in conjunction with addiction.

psychotomimetic—a state that imitates a state of psychosis. Usually associated with the hallucinogens.

psychotropic—changing the state of consciousness.

pusher—one who sells drugs.

Q

Quaalude—methaqualone. Frequently abused drug. Associated both with getting high and increased sexual experience.

quarter moon—hashish.

R

rainbows—Tuinal capsules, a form of barbiturate.

red devils—Seconal capsules, a form of barbiturate.

reefer—a marijuana joint.

resin—the sticky oil secreted by the marijuana plant.

rig—the paraphernalia for injecting drugs.

Ritalin—a stimulant drug related to amphetamines. Used in treating hyperactivity in children.

roach clip, roach holder—holder for a marijuana joint.

rush—the initial feeling just following the ingestion or injection of a drug.

S

scars—needle tracks left from injecting a drug into veins.

scheduled drugs—those drugs that are listed under the Controlled Substances Act.

schmack—drugs, especially heroin.

score—buy narcotics.

script—a narcotics prescription.

Seconal—a barbiturate.

set up—to arrange to have a person arrested for drugs; *setup*—combination of ups and downs (barbiturates and amphetamines).

shooting gallery—place where addicts go to shoot up.

skin popping—injecting drugs under the skin or into the muscle.

smack—heroin.

snappers—small bottles of amyl nitrite.

sniffing—inhaling a substance, usually heroin or cocaine.

snorting—same as sniffing.

snow—cocaine.

soaper—methaqualone.

soft drugs—nonnarcotic drugs, some of which are addicting.

Sopor—methaqualone.

spaced—in a state of altered consciousness. Similar to *spaced out*.

speed—amphetamines.

speedball—heroin and cocaine or amphetamine that is injected.

speed freak—heavy user of speed (amphetamines).

star dust—cocaine.

stash place—where drugs are kept or hidden.

stick—marijuana cigarette.

stimulants—drugs that stimulate the central nervous system.

stoned—in a drugged state of euphoria. Similar to *high*.

straight—sober, not using drugs.
street—refers to the drug-using world.
strung out—being addicted.

T

Talwin—a synthetic opiod pain reliever. Can cause addiction.
tea—marijuana.
terpin hydrate—nonnarcotic cough suppressant.
tetrahydro-cannabinol (THC)—the active ingredient in marijuana. It is responsible for the euphoric effect.
Thorazine—major antipsychotic tranquilizer. Used in the treatment of schizophrenia and for drug-induced psychosis.
toke—to smoke marijuana.
tolerance—built-up resistance to a drug's effect. Responsible for addiction.
tracks—needle marks from injecting drugs intravenously.
trip—take a hallucinogen.
turn on—introduce someone to drugs. To be high on drugs.

U

up—a state of being high or happy.
uppers, ups—amphetamine pills.
using—using drugs.

V

Valium—a minor tranquilizer mainly used as an antianxiety drug.
violated—arrested for violation of parole or probation.

W

wake-up—first shot of drugs in the morning.
waste—use up, destroy or kill.

weed—marijuana.

white stuff—heroin. Occasionally cocaine.

wiped out—very intoxicated on a chemical.

wired—addicted or highly intoxicated.

withdrawal—physical discomfort associated with stopping the use of a drug that a person is addicted to. Can occur when dosage is lessened.

Y

yellows, yellow jackets—Nembutal, a barbiturate.

yen—a craving, such as a craving for drugs.

yohimbe root—supposedly an aphrodisiac, but doubtful.

Z

Zigzag—a favorite rolling paper for marijuana cigarettes.

zonked—very high on drugs or passed out from drugs.

Resources

HOSPITAL TREATMENT

Jason D. Baron, M.D.
Drug Abuse Programs of America, Inc. (DAPA)
P.O. Box 5487
Pasadena, Tex. 77505 (713) 479-8440

Packet of articles on drug-related topics—$5.00.
Literature about DAPA Treatment Programs—free.

PREVENTION GROUPS

American Council on Marijuana (ACM)
767 Fifth Ave.
New York, N.Y. 10022
Marijuana Today (revised edition), by George K. Russell, Ph.D. (Myrin Institute). A compilation of medical findings for the layman. $3.00.

Keep Off the Grass: A Scientist's Documented Account of Marijuana's Destructive Effects, by Gabriel Nahas, M.D. (Pergamon Press). The marijuana story from 1969 to 1980, with emphasis on harmful physical effects. $9.50.

Twelve Is Too Old, by Peggy Man (Doubleday). The first novel for teens and preteens to deal realistically with the pot scene. Also contains medical information. $7.95.

Marijuana: Biological Effects and Social Implications. Reports of 12 noted psychiatrists, physicians, and organizers of parents groups. $5.00.

Citizens for Informed Choices on Marijuana (CICOM)
300 Broad St.
Stamford, Conn. 06901
Four booklets with methods to combat marijuana, plus 1-year membership. $10.00.

Committees of Correspondence
P.O. Box 1590, Cathedral Station
New York, N.Y. 10025
Ideas for communicating your concerns by letter and telephone. Special drug issue monthly. $7.00/yr.

Executive Information Resources
Box 611
Wellington, Kan. 67152
Unedited cassette tapes of the general sessions of the Grass Roots Conference on Grass held in Washington. Tapes are priced at $6.40 each or $35.00 for a complete set of 7 tapes. Prices include shipping.

Families in Action
P.O. Box 15053
Atlanta, Ga. 30333
Manual to help organize your community to combat the drug culture. $10.00. Quarterly newsletter which includes latest information on the drug scene at state, national and international levels. $3.00.

Marijuana Under the Microscope
  Drug Enforcement Administration
  Preventive Program Section
  Washington, D.C. 20537
  Articles on health hazards and drug paraphernalia.
  Single copies free.

Medical Education and Research Foundation
  Box 2166
  Indianapolis, Ind., 46202
  *Marijuana: The Myth of Harmlessness Goes Up in
  Smoke,* by Peggy Mann. Booklet with the latest medical information on the effects of marijuana on the
  brain, male and female reproductive system, pulmonary system, immune system, and cellular impairment; plus many black-and-white and color pictures
  showing pot-impaired brain cells, sperm, ova, etc.
  (Reprint of two-part *Saturday Evening Post* article).
  One to 9 copies, $1.00 each; 10 or more, $.60 each;
  100 or more $.50 each; 1000 or more, $.20 each.

Minicourses
  4290 Raintree Lane NW
  Atlanta, Ga. 30327
  Six-unit teaching manual, *Drug Abuse and the Growing Child,* for third through eighth grades (for schools,
  homes, and agencies). $10.00. Cassette with narra-
  tion, plus 80 color slides showing youth drug subculture, plus prevention methods. $46.75.

Narcotics Education, Inc.
  6830 Laurel Street, N.W.
  Washington, D.C. 20012
  Six question-and-answer booklets on marijuana and
  PCP, and *Parents' Guide to Drug Abuse,* $2.00. *Listen*
  (magazine for teens) special issue on drugs, $1.00.
  March, 1980.

National Drug Abuse Foundation
   6500 Randall Place
   Falls Church, Va. 22044
   Information on common drugs abused, recommended
   reading. $2.00.

National Federation of Parents for Drug Free Youth
   P.O. Box 57217
   Pennsylvania Ave.
   Washington, D.C. 20037
   NFP Starter Kit. $1.00.

National Institute on Drug Abuse
   P.O. Box 2305
   Rockville, Md. 20852
   Parents, Peers, and Pot, a 98-page paperback with advice on coping with adolescent drug use, based on the
   experience of parents who successfully dealt with the
   problem. Single copy free.

   For Parents Only: What Kids Think About Marijuana,
   a 30-minute 16mm film available on free loan to parent
   groups and adult community organizations (specify
   date needed). Contact Modern Talking Picture Service, 5000 Park Street North, St. Petersburg, Florida
   33709. With film comes discussion guidebook and 25
   free copies of *For Parents Only* booklet.

   *For Parents Only: What You Need to Know About
   Marijuana,* a 20-page booklet. Single copy free.

Phoenix House
   164 West 74th St.
   New York, N.Y. 10023
   Free information on drugs, plus advice on school programs.

Prevention Materials Institute
    P.O. Box 152
    Lafayette, Calif. 94549
    Communicating About Drugs, for parents and teachers. $1.75.

PRIDE (Parent Resources and Information on Drug Education)
    University Plaza
    Georgia State University
    Atlanta, Ga. 30303
    Information on drugs, including action plan for parents and their school community. $5.00. Quarterly newsletter. $2.00.

STOP (Society to Oppose Pot)
    P.O. Box 6772
    Silver Spring, Md. 20906
    Booklet and briefing by lawyers on how to muster local political pressure to influence elected officials in reference to antidrug legislation. $3.00.

Texans' War on Drugs
    Write to DARE
    7800 Shoal Creek Blvd., 381-W
    Austin, Tex. 78757

Texas Department of Community Affairs, State Program on Drug Abuse
    P.O. Box 13166, Capital Station
    Austin, Tex. 78711.
    "Drugs and Drug Abuse."

RECOMMENDED READING FOR PROFESSIONALS

Alcohol and Illicit Drug Use.
National Institute for Drug Abuse Services Research Report. Superintendent of Documents, U.S. Government Printing Office. Washington, D.C. 20402. 1977.

Alternative Pursuits for America's 3rd Century.
A resource book on new perceptions, processes, and programs. National Institute for Drug Abuse, 5600 Fishers Lane, Rockville, Md. 20857. 1974.

Annotated Bibliography of Papers from the Addiction Research Center 1935–1975.
U.S. Dept. of Health, Education, and Welfare; U.S. Public Health Service; Alcohol, Drug Abuse and Mental Health Administration. National Institute for Drug Abuse, 5600 Fishers Lane, Rockville, Md. 20857. 1978.

The Behavioral Aspects of Smoking.
Krasnegor, N.A. National Institute for Drug Abuse, 5600 Fishers Lane, Rockville, Md. 20857. 1979.

Behavioral Tolerance: Research and Treatment Implications.
Research Monograph Series 18. N.A. Krasnegor, ed. U.S. Dept. of Health, Education, and Welfare; U.S. Public Health Service; Alcohol, Drug Abuse and Mental Health Administration. National Institute for Drug Abuse, 5600 Fishers Lane, Rockville, Md. Jan., 1978.

Catlin, D.H. *A Guide to Urine Testing for Drugs of Abuse.*
Executive Office of the President. Special Action Office for Drug Abuse Prevention. 726 Jackson Place, N.W., Washington, D.C. 20500. 1973.

CNS Depressants. Technical Papers No. 1.
National Clearinghouse for Drug Abuse Information.
National Institute for Drug Abuse, 11400 Rockville
Pike, Rockville, Md. 20852. 1974.

Criminal Charge and Drug Use Patterns of Arrestees in the District of Columbia.
Kozel, M.S., and DuPont, R.L. National Institute for
Drug Abuse Technical Paper. National Institute for
Drug Abuse, 11400 Rockville Pike, Rockville, Md.
20852. 1977.

Developing and Using a Vocational Training and Educational Resource Manual.
National Institute for Drug Abuse Services Research
Report. Superintendent of Documents. U.S. Government Printing Office. Washington, D.C. 20402. 1977.

Drug Treatment Histories for a Sample of Drug Users in DARP.
National Institute for Drug Abuse Services Research
Report. DHEW Publications No. 78-634. Superintendent of Documents, U.S. Government Printing Office, Washington, D.C. 20402. 1978.

Drug Treatment in New York City and Washington, D.C.
Service Research Monograph Series, National Institute for Drug Abuse, 5600 Fishers Lane, Rockville,
Md. 20857. 1977.

Drug Users and the Criminal Justice System.
Research Issues 18. Austin, G.A., and Lettieri, D.J.,
eds. National Institute for Drug Abuse, 5600 Fishers
Lane, Rockville, Md. 20857. June, 1977.

Drugs and Crime.
Research Issues 17. Austin, G.A., and Lettieri, D.J.,
eds. U.S. Dept. of Health, Education, and Welfare;
U.S. Public Health Service; Alcohol, Drug Abuse and

Mental Health Administration. National Institute for Drug Abuse, 5600 Fishers Lane, Rockville, Md. 20857. March, 1977.

Drugs and Driving.
Research Monograph Series 11. Willette, R.E., ed. U.S. Public Health Service; Alcohol, Drug Abuse and Mental Health Administration. National Institute for Drug Abuse, 5600 Fishers Lane, Rockville, Md. 20857. March, 1977.

Drugs and Minorities.
Research Issues 21. Austin, G.A., et al., eds. U.S. Dept. of Health, Education, and Welfare; U.S. Public Health Service; Alcohol, Drug Abuse and Mental Health Administration. National Institute for Drug Abuse, 5600 Fishers Lane, Rockville, Md. 20857. 1977.

Drugs and Pregnancy.
Research Issues 5. Ferguson, P., Lennox, T., and Letticri, D.J., eds. National Institute for Drug Abuse, 5600 Fishers Lane, Rockville, Md. 20857. November, 1974.

The Epidemiology of Heroin and Other Narcotics.
National Institute for Drug Abuse Research Monograph Series 16. Rittenhouse, J.D., ed. U.S. Dept. of Health, Education, and Welfare; U.S. Public Health Service; Alcohol, Drug Abuse and Mental Health Administration. National Institute for Drug Abuse, 5600 Fishers Lane, Rockville, Md. 20857. 1977.

An Evaluation of the California Civil Addict Program.
McGlothin, W. H.; Anglin, M.D.; and Wilson, B.D. U.S. Dept. of Health, Education, and Welfare; U.S. Public Health Service; Alcohol, Drug Abuse and Mental Health Administration. National Institute for Drug Abuse, 5600 Fishers Lane, Rockville, Md. 20857. 1977.

Followup Evaluation of Drug Abuse Treatment: A Summary Report.
National Institute for Drug Abuse Services Research Report. U.S. Dept. of Health, Education, and Welfare Publication No. (ADM) 79-765. Superintendent of Documents, U.S. Government Printing Office, Washington, D.C. 20402. 1978.

Intervention Drug Use.
Research Issues 23. Austin, G.A., Macari, M.A., and Lettieri, D.J., eds. U.S. Dept. of Health, Education, and Welfare; U.S. Public Health Service; Alcohol, Drug Abuse and Mental Health Administration. National Institute for Drug Abuse, 5600 Fishers Lane, Rockville, Md. 20857. 1978.

Marks, J. *The Benzodiazepines; Use, Overuse, Misuse, Abuse.* Baltimore, Md.: University Park Press, 1978.

Medical Treatment for Complications of Polydrug Abuse. Treatment Manual 1.
U.S. Dept. of Health, Education, and Welfare; U.S. Public Health Service; Alcohol, Drug Abuse, and Mental Health Administration. National Institute for Drug Abuse, 5600 Fishers Lane, Rockville, Md. 20857. 1978.

Narcotic Antagonists: The Search for Long-Acting Preparations.
R. Willette, National Institute for Drug Abuse, 5600 Fishers Lane, Rockville, Md. 20857. 1975.

National Manpower and Training System.
Source Book. National Institute for Drug Abuse, 5600 Fishers Lane, Rockville, Md. 20857.

Nonurban Drug Abuse Programs: A Descriptive Study.
National Institute for Drug Abuse Services Research Report. U.S. Dept. of Health, Education, and Wel-

fare Publication No. (ADM) 78-636. 1978. Superintendent of Documents, U.S. Government Printing
Office, Washington, D.C. 20402. 1978.

Perspectives on the History of Psychoactive Substance Use.
Research Issues 24. Austin, G.A. U.S. Dept. of
Health, Education, and Welfare; U.S. Public Health
Service; Alcohol, Drug Abuse and Mental Health Ad-
ministration. National Institute for Drug Abuse, 5600
Fishers Lane, Rockville, Md. 20857. June, 1978.

Psychosocial Characteristics of Drug-Abusing Women.
Burt, M.R. U.S. Dept. of Health, Education, and
Welfare; U.S. Public Health Service; Alcohol, Drug
Abuse and Mental Health Administration. National
Institute for Drug Abuse, 5600 Fishers Lane, Rock-
ville, Md. 20857. 1979.

*Referral Strategies for Polydrug Abusers. Treatment Man-
ual 3.*
U.S. Dept. of Health, Education, and Welfare; U.S.
Public Health Service; Alcohol, Drug Abuse, and
Mental Health Administration. National Institute for
Drug Abuse, 5600 Fishers Lane, Rockville, Md.
20857. 1977.

*Report of the Task Force on Comparability in Survey Re-
search on Drugs.*
Rittenhouse, J.D. National Institute for Drug Abuse
Technical paper. National Institute for Drug Abuse,
5600 Fishers Lane, Rockville, Md. 20857. 1978.

Research Issues Update, 1978.
Research Issues 22, Austin, G.A., Macari, M.A., and
lettieri, D.J., eds. U.S. Dept. of Health, Education,
and Welfare; U.S. Public Health Service; Alchol,
Drug Abuse and Mental Health Administration. National Institute for Drug Abuse, 5600 Fishers Lane,
Rockville, Md. 1979.

Review of Inhalants: Euphoria to Dysfunction.
Research Monograph Series 15. Sharp, C.W., and Brehm, M.L., eds. U.S. Dept. of Health, Education, and Welfare; U.S. Public Health Service; Alcohol, Drug Abuse and Mental Health Administration. National Institute for Drug Abuse, 5600 Fishers Lane, Rockville, Md. 20857. October, 1977.

Robins, L.N. *The Vietnam Drug User Returns, Special Action Office Monograph.* Series A, Number 2, National Institute for Drug Abuse, 5600 Fishers Lane, Rockville, Md. 20857 1974.

Schukit, M.A. *Drug and Alcohol Abuse.* Plenum Medicine Book Company, 1979.

Securing Employment for Ex-Drug Abusers: An Overview of Jobs.
National Institute for Drug Abuse Services Research Report. Superintendent of Documents, U.S. Government Printing Office, Washington, D.C. 20402. 1977.

Senay, E.C., et al. *The Primary Physician's Guide to Drug Abuse Treatment.*
State University of New York, 450 Clarkson Ave., Brooklyn, N.Y. 11203. June, 1979.

Skills Training and Employment for Ex-Addicts in Washington, D.C.
A Report on Treatment. National Institute for Drug Abuse Services Research Report. U.S. Dept. of Health, Education, and Welfare Publication No. (ADM) 78-694. Superintendent of Documents, U.S. Government Printing Office, Washington, D.C. 20402. 1978.

A Study of Legal Drug Use by Older Americans.
Gattman, D., U.S. Dept. of Health, Education, and Welfare; U.S. Public Health Service; Alcohol, Drug

Abuse and Mental Health Administration. National Institute for Drug Abuse, 5600 Fishers Lane, Rockville, Md. 20857. 1977.

Toward a Heroin Problem Index—An Analytical Model for Drug Abuse Indicators. Person, P.H., et al. National Institute for Drug Abuse, 5600 Fishers Lane, Rockville, Md. 20857. 1978.

The Wildcat Experiment: An Early Test of Supported Work in Drug Abuse Rehabilitation. Friedman, L.N. Vera Institute of Justice. U.S. Dept. of Health, Education, and Welfare; U.S. Public Health Service; Alcohol, Drug Abuse and Mental Health Administration. National Institute for Drug Abuse, 5600 Fishers Lane, Rockville, Md. 20857. 1978.

Withdrawal from Methadone Maintenance: Rate of Withdrawal and Expectation.
National Institute for Drug Abuse Services Research Report. Superintendent of Documents, U.S. Government Printing Office, Washington, D.C. 20402. 1977.

RECOMMENDED GENERAL READING

A Cocaine Bibliography—nonannotated.
Research Issues 8. Phillips, J.L., and Wynne, R.D. National Institute for Drug Abuse, 11400 Rockville Pike, Rockville, Md. 20852. November, 1974.

A Family Response to the Drug Problem.
U.S. Dept. of Health, Education, and Welfare; U.S. Public Health Service; Alcohol, Drug Abuse and Mental Health Administration. National Institute for Drug Abuse, 11400 Rockville Pike, Rockville, Md. 20852. 1976.

Alpert, R., and Cohen, S. *L.S.D.* New York: The New American Library, 1966.

A Woman's Choice: Deciding About Drugs.
National Institute for Drug Abuse; U.S. Dept. of Health, Education, and Welfare; U.S. Public Health Service; Alcohol, Drug Abuse and Mental Health Administration. National Institute for Drug Abuse, 5600 Fishers Lane, Rockville, Md. 20857. 1979.

Baron, J. D., and Mann, P. "Kids and Drugs. New Facts, New Fears, New Hope." *Family Circle*, pp. 46–52, April 7, 1982.

Behavioral Analysis in Treatment of Substance Abuse.
Krasnegor, N.A. Research Issues 25, National Institute for Drug Abuse, 5600 Fishers Lane, Rockville, Md. 20857. June, 1979.

Bromwell, S. "How I Got My Daughter to Stop Smoking Pot." *Good Housekeeping*, March, 1979.

Cocaine: 1977.
National Institute for Drug Abuse Research Monograph #13. Peterson, R.C., and Stillman, R.C., eds. U.S. Dept. of Health, Education, and Welfare; U.S. Public Health Service; Alcohol, Drug Abuse and Mental Health Administration. National Institute for Drug Abuse, 5600 Fishers Lane, Rockville, Md. 20857. May, 1977.

Consequences of Alcohol and Marijuana Use.
Rittenhouse, J.D. National Institute for Drug Abuse. 1979.

Drug Users and Driving Behavior.
Research Issues 20. Austin, G.A., et al., eds. U.S. Dept. of Health, Education, and Welfare; U.S. Public Health Service; Alcohol, Drug Abuse and Mental

Health Administration. National Institute for Drug Abuse, 5600 Fishers Lane, Rockville, Md. 20852. June, 1977.

Drugs and Death.
Research Issues 6. Ferguson, P., Lennox, T., and Lettieri, D.J. National Institute for Drug Abuse, 5600 Fishers Lane, Rockville, Md. 20852. November, 1974.

Drugs and Psychopathology.
Research Issues 19. Austin, G.A., et al. National Institute for Drug Abuse, 5600 Fishers Lane, Rockville, Md. June, 1977.

Drugs and Sex.
Research Issues 2. Ferguson, P., Lennox, T., and Lettieri, D.J., eds. U.S. Dept. of Health, Education, and Welfare; U.S. Public Health Service; Alcohol, Drug Abuse and Mental Health Administration. National Institute for Drug Abuse, 11400 Rockville Pike, Rockville, Md. 20852. 1977.

Drugs and the Nation's High School Students.
1979 Highlights. Johnston, L.D., Bachman, J.G., and O'Malley, P.M. The University of Michigan Institute for Social Research. National Institute for Drug Abuse, Division of Research, 5600 Fishers Lane, Rockville, Md. 20857. 1979.

Family Therapy: A Summary of Selected Literature.
U.S. Dept. of Health, Education, and Welfare; U.S. Public Health Service; Alcohol, Drug Abuse and Mental Health Administration. National Institute for Drug Abuse, 5600 Fishers Lane, Rockville, Md. 20852. 1980.

Fort, Joel, M.D. *Alcohol: Our Biggest Drug Problem.* New York: McGraw-Hill Book Co., 1973.

Hart, R.H. *Bitter Grass—The Cruel Truth About Marijuana.*
Psychoneurologia Press, P.O. Box 7542, Shawness Mission, Kan., 1980.

Highlights from Drugs and the Class of '78: Behaviors, Attitudes, and Recent National Trends.
U.S. Dept. of Health, Education, and Welfare; U.S. Public Health Service; Alcohol, Drug Abuse and Mental Health Administration. National Institute for Drug Abuse, 5600 Fishers Lane, Rockville, Md. 20857. 1979.

Janeczek, Curtis L. *Marijuana: Time for a Closer Look.*
Healthstar Publications, P.O. Box 8426, Columbia, Ohio, 43201. $4.95.

Mann, Peggy. *Marijuana Update.* Reprints, *Reader's Digest,* Pleasantville, N.Y. 10570, or phone toll free, 800-431-1726. "Digest Size" booklet (24 pages) with four articles on health hazards of marijuana from *Reader's Digest* ("Marijuana Alert I and II" and "Marijuana Driving"). Single copies, $1.25; 10 copies, $7.00; 25 copies, $15.00; 50 copies, $25.00; 100 copies, $40.00; 500 copies, $150.00; 1000 copies, $200.00.

Mann, Peggy. "The Case Against Marijuana."
Family Circle, February, 1979.

Marijuana and Health. 8th Annual Report to the U.S. Congress. National Institute for Drug Abuse, 5600 Fishers Lane, Rockville, Md. 20857.

Marijuana Research Findings: 1976.
Research Monograph Series 14. U.S. Dept. of Health, Education, and Welfare; U.S. Public Health Service; Alcohol, Drug Abuse and Mental Health Administration. National Institute for Drug Abuse, 5600 Fishers Lane, Rockville, Md. 20857.

Marijuana Research Findings: 1980.
 Research Monograph Series 31. U.S. Dept. of Health,
 Education, and Welfare; U.S. Public Health Service;
 Alcohol, Drug Abuse and Mental Health Administra-
 tion. National Institute for Drug Abuse, 5600 Fishers
 Lane, Rockville, Md. 20857. June, 1980.

"Mr. Pecksniff's Horse? (Psychodynamics in Compulsive
 Drug Use)."
 Wurmser, L., *Psychodynamics of Drug Dependence*,
 National Institute for Drug Abuse Research Mono-
 graph Series 12, pp. 36–72. May, 1977.

Nahas, G.G., and Frick, H.C. II. *Drug Abuse in the Modern World*. Elmsford, N.Y.: Pergamon Press, 1980.

Neff, P. *Tough Love*. New York: Abingdon Press, 1982.

PCP—Phencyclidine Abuse: An Appraisal.
 Research Monograph Series 21. Petersen, R.C., and
 Stillman, R.C., eds. U.S. Dept. of Health, Education,
 and Welfare; U.S. Public Health Service; Alcohol,
 Drug Abuse and Mental Health Administration. Na-
 tional Institute for Drug Abuse, 5600 Fishers Lane,
 Rockville, Md. 20857. August, 1978.

Pot Safari
 By Peggy Mann. Foxrun Press, P.O. Box 1590, Cathedral Station, New York, N.Y. 10025. $3.00. Contains
 the newest and some of the most startling information
 ever published on marijuana. Writer Peggy Mann,
 who has written on the subject for *Reader's Digest*,
 Washington Post, Ladies' Home Journal and other
 magazines, took a "pot safari" to spend several days
 with each of the top marijuana researchers in the
 United States. This booklet is the result, with striking
 photographs.

Ray, O. *Drugs, Society, and Human Behavior*. St. Louis, Mo.: C.V. Mosby Co., 1978.

Research on Smoking Behavior.
Research Monograph Series 17. U.S. Dept. of Health, Education, and Welfare; U.S. Public Health Service; Alcohol, Drug Abuse and Mental Health Administration. National Institute for Drug Abuse, 5600 Fishers Lane, Rockville, Md. 20857. December, 1977.

Ropp, R. S. *Drugs and the Mind*. New York: Delacorte Press, 1976.

Schultes, R. E. *Hallucinogenic Plants*. New York: Golden Press, 1976.

Silver, Gary. *The Dope Chronicles, 1850–1950*. New York: Harper & Row, 1979.

Sparks, B. *Jay's Journal*. New York: Dell Publishing, 1979.

The International Challenge of Drug Abuse.
Research Monograph 19. Petersen, R. C., ed. U.S. Dept. of Health, Education, and Welfare; U.S. Public Health Service; Alcohol, Drug Abuse and Mental Health Administration. National Institute for Drug Abuse, 5600 Fishers Lane, Rockville, Md. 20857. 1978.

Theories on Drug Abuse: Selected Contemporary Perspectives.
Research Monograph. Lettieri, D.J., Sayers, M., and Pearson, H.W., eds. U.S. Dept. of Health, Education, and Welfare; U.S. Public Health Service; Alcohol, Drug Abuse and Mental Health Administration. National Institute for Drug Abuse, 5600 Fishers Lane, Rockville, Md. 20857. March, 1980.

The Therapeutic Community.
De Leon, G., and Beschner, G.M. National Institute for Drug Abuse, 5600 Fishers Lane, Rockville, Md. 20857.

"Time to Change Attitudes on Marijuana."
Patient Care, pp. 182–216, April 30, 1978.

Turner, Carlton, and Waller, Coy, and associates.
Marijuana: An Annotated Bibliography. Volume 1. Macmillan Information, 200-D Brown Street, Riverside, N.J.

Voth, H. *How to Get Your Child Off Marijuana.*
Citizens for Informed Choices on Marijuana (CICOM), 300 Broad St., Stamford, Conn. 06901. $3.00.

THE DRUG ABUSE PROGRAMS OF AMERICA (DAPA)

P.O. Box 5487
Pasadena, Texas 77505
(713) 479-8440

INDEX